Manual of
3D ECHOCARDIOGRAPHY

System requirement:

- Operating system—Windows XP or above
- Web browser—Internet Explorer 8 or above, Mozilla Firefox and Safari
- Essential plugins—Java & Flash player
  - Facing problems in viewing content—it may be your system does not have java enabled.
  - If Videos don't show up—it may be the system requires Flash player or need to manage flash setting
  - You can test java and flash by using the links from the troubleshoot section of the CD/DVD.
- Learn more about flash setting from the link in the troubleshoot section.

Accompanying CD/DVD-ROM is playable only in Computer and not in DVD player.

CD/DVD has Autorun function—it may take few seconds to load on your computer. If it does not works for you then follow the steps below to access the contents manually:

- Click on my computer
- Select the CD/DVD drive and click open/explore—this will show list of files in the CD/DVD
- Find and double click file—"launch.html"

DVD Contents

1. Introduction to 3D Echocardiography
   Dr RA Janarthanan MD DM
2. Introduction to 3D Echo Techniques
   Dr V Amuthan MD DM FACC
3. Proceedings of Workshop on 3D Echocardiography in Device Closure for (Aterial Septal Defects) ASD
4. Proceedings of Workshop on 3D Echo in Balloon Mitral Valvuloplasty

Manual of 3D ECHOCARDIOGRAPHY

Editor

V Amuthan MD DM FACC FIAE FCSI
The Emeritus Professor
Department of Cardiology
The Tamil Nadu Dr MGR Medical University
Chennai, Tamil Nadu

Formerly Professor and Head
Department of Cardiology
Madurai Medical College and Government Rajaji Hospital
Madurai, Tamil Nadu

Consultant Cardiologist
Vadamalayan Hospitals
Madurai, Tamil Nadu

Consultant Cardiologist
Jeyalakshmi Heart Centre
Madurai, Tamil Nadu, India

Foreword
M Srinivasan

JAYPEE BROTHERS MEDICAL PUBLISHERS (P) LTD

New Delhi • Panama City • London • Dhaka • Kathmandu

Jaypee Brothers Medical Publishers (P) Ltd

Headquarters

Jaypee Brothers Medical Publishers (P) Ltd
4838/24, Ansari Road, Daryaganj
New Delhi 110 002, India
Phone: +91-11-43574357
Fax: +91-11-43574314
Email: jaypee@jaypeebrothers.com

Overseas Offices

J.P. Medical Ltd
83 Victoria Street, London
SW1H 0HW (UK)
Phone: +44-2031708910
Fax: +02-03-0086180
Email: info@jpmedpub.com

Jaypee-Highlights Medical Publishers Inc.
City of Knowledge, Bld. 237, Clayton
Panama City, Panama
Phone: +507-301-0496
Fax: +507-301-0499
Email: cservice@jphmedical.com

Jaypee Brothers Medical Publishers (P) Ltd
17/1-B Babar Road, Block-B, Shaymali
Mohammadpur, Dhaka-1207
Bangladesh
Mobile: +08801912003485
Email: jaypeedhaka@gmail.com

Jaypee Brothers Medical Publishers (P) Ltd
Shorakhute, Kathmandu
Nepal
Phone: +00977-9841528578
Email: jaypee.nepal@gmail.com

Website: www.jaypeebrothers.com
Website: www.jaypeedigital.com

Inquiries for bulk sales may be solicited at: jaypee@jaypeebrothers.com

Manual of 3D Echocardiography

First Edition: **2013**

ISBN 978-93-5025-586-5

Printed at Ajanta Offset & Packaging Ltd., New Delhi

Dedicated to

My wife Rajammal

and

My children

RVA Ananth and RVA Arthy Jeya

Contributors

A Jegadeeswari MD
Senior Resident
Department of Cardiology
Madurai Medical College
Madurai, Tamil Nadu, India

Balu Vaidyanathan MD DM
Clinical Professor
Department of Cardiology
Amrita Insititute of Medical Sciences
Ernakulam, Kerala, India

C Balachandran MD DM
Assistant Professor
Department of Cardiology
Thirunelveli Medical College
Thirunelveli, Tamil Nadu, India

Girish S Shirali MD
Department of Pediatric Cardiology
Medical University of South Carolina
USA

GS Siva Kumar MD DM
Assistant Professor
Department of Cardiology
Madurai Medical College
Madurai, Tamil Nadu, India

John M Simpson MD
Professor
Department of Imaging Sciences
Evelina Children Hospital
St Thomas Hospital, London, UK

N Ganesan MD DM
Assistant Professor
Department of Cardiology
Madurai Medical College
Madurai, Tamil Nadu, India

P Ashok Kumar MD DM
Assistant Professor
Department of Cardiology
Thanjavur Medical College
Thanjavur, Tamil Nadu, India

RA Janarthanan MD DM
Professor and Head
Department of Cardiology
Madurai Medical College
Madurai, Tamil Nadu, India

R Alagesan MD DM
Professor and Head
Department of Cardiology (Retd)
Madras Medical College
Chennai, Tamil Nadu, India

Raman Krishna Kumar MD DM
Professor
Department of Cardiology
Amirtha Institute of Medical Sciences
Ernakulam, Kerala, India

R Aravazhi MD
Senior Resident
Department of Cardiology
Madurai Medical College
Madurai, Tamil Nadu, India

S Balasubramanian MD DM
Professor and Head
Department of Cardiology
Government Mohan Kumaramangalam
Medical College, Salem, Tamil Nadu, India

S Naina Mohamed MD DM
Assistant Professor
Department of Cardiology
Madurai Medical College
Madurai, Tamil Nadu, India

SR Veeramani MD DM
Assistant Professor
Department of Cardiology
Madurai Medical College
Madurai, Tamil Nadu, India

V Amuthan MD DM FACC FIAE FCSI
The Emeritus Professor
Department of Cardiology
The Tamil Nadu Dr MGR Medical University
Chennai, Tamil Nadu

Formerly Professor and Head
Department of Cardiology
Madurai Medical College and Government Rajaji Hospital
Madurai, Tamil Nadu

Consultant Cardiologist
Vadamalayan Hospitals
Madurai, Tamil Nadu

Consultant Cardiologist
Jeyalakshmi Heart Centre
Madurai, Tamil Nadu, India

Foreword

The twentieth century witnessed great leaps in diagnostic imaging, Echocardiography, CT imaging and MRI to name a few. Though introduced by Elder in 1953, Echocardiography was a curiosity like Apex Cardiography and Balisto Cardiogram in the formative years.

When M-mode echocardiogram was refined in the early seventies and with the widespread cooperation of industry, it came to clinical arena. Its usefulness in early stages was restricted to the diagnosis of pericardial effusion and valvular heart diseases.

Then, two major breakthroughs came in the early eighties—Real-time 2D imaging and integration of Doppler echo, and later real-time color flow too was added to the armamentarium. With this, we had a tool with high diagnostic accuracy both in terms of specificity and sensitivity. For a brief period, invasive hemodynamics was surpassed—only to re-emerge after development of transcatheter therapeutics. The next major advance is real-time 3D echocardiography with integration of color flow mapping.

The diagnostic accuracy with 3D echo equals surgical exploration and autopsy studies. It is also emerging as an important, useful tool in the assessment of percutaneous cardiovascular interventions, especially in the treatment of septal defects and valvular heart disease.

Dr Amuthan has taken great efforts to put together the advances in 3D echo in a beautiful comprehensive monograph with the help of pioneers in the field. It is a commendable effort by him. Dr Amuthan always looks forward. I hope the monograph and the symposium will enlighten the postgraduates, consultants and novice in this field like me. It gives me pleasure to share a few thoughts as foreword. It is easy to write foreword than to contribute scientific material. Hence, I have chosen this job.

I wish all success to Dr Amuthan's endeavors.

M Srinivasan MD DM
Senior Interventional Cardiologist
Vadamalayan Hospital,
Madurai, Tamil Nadu, India

Preface

It gives me immense pleasure to bring out this *Manual of 3D Echocardiography*. This book is aimed at students of echocardiography, cardiologists and physicians performing basic two-dimensional and color Doppler echocardiography. The book has been made possible with enormous grants from Dr Pugazhagiri Vadamalayan, Managing Director, Vadamalayan Heart Foundation and Philips India Limited.

There is an initial chapter on 3D echocardiogram by Professor Dr R Alagesan. This is followed by a chapter fully dedicated on "How to perform 3D echocardiography" by the uninitiated. Tips and tricks of the trade have been given as a separate table. This is followed by 3 chapters on valvular heart disease. There is a dedicated chapter on Coronary Artery Disease emphasizing the need for calculation of 3D regional wall motion abnormalities and ejection fraction. There has been a dedicated chapter on congenital heart disease by Professor Girish S Shirali, with permission from Annals of Pediatric Cardiology. Professor Dr Raman Krishna Kumar has written a chapter on Interventional Device Closure in Atrial Septal Defects which has been reproduced with permission from JACC imaging. There is a separate chapter on 3D Transthoracic ecocardiography (TTE) and Transesophageal ecocardiography (TEE) in interventions. Finally, we have taken great efforts to reproduce some of the interesting 3D echo clippings as an atlas.

I take this opportunity to thank our medical superintendent Professor Dr SM Siva Kumar, who has helped our department in all our endeavors.

My solid work in cardiology would not have been possible without encouragement and inspiration from my teachers, Professor Dr T Sakthivel and Profesor Dr N Kasirajan. I have the esteemed pleasure of support from my Associate Professor Dr RA Janarthanan, Assistant Professors Dr S Balasubramanian, Dr S Naina Mohamed, Dr N Ganesan, Dr GS Siva Kumar and my postgraduates Dr SR Veeramani, Dr P Ashok Kumar, Dr R Aravazhi, Dr R Sampath Kumar, Dr RR Saravanan and Dr A Jegadeeswari.

My great inspiration for my higher studies in cardiology would not have been possible without my parents Professor R Vivekanandan, and Mrs Jeyalakshmi, and my brother Dr RV Asokan, MD.

I dedicate my work to my beloved wife and my children.

V Amuthan

Contents

CHAPTER 1

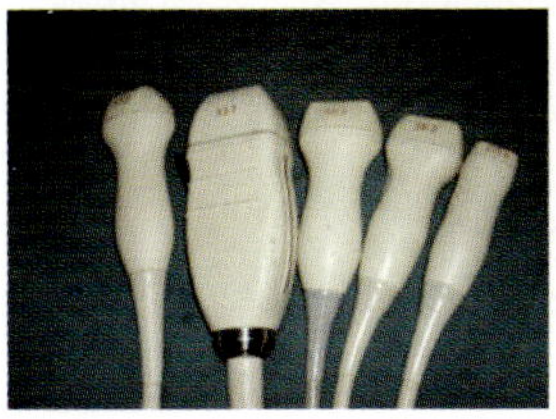

Real-Time Three-Dimensional Echocardiography

R Alagesan, V Amuthan

INTRODUCTION

Conventional two-dimensional (2D) echocardiography requires mental conceptualization of a series of multiple orthogonal planar or tomographic images into an imaginary multidimensional reconstruction for better understanding of complex intracardiac structures and their spatial relation with surroundings. The emerging three-dimensional (3D) echocardiographic imaging technique is a major step ahead toward the final goal of complete visualization and comprehensive assessment of cardiac anatomy, physiology, pathomorphology and pathophysiology in real-time, which could potentially facilitate image interpretation and reduce inter-observer variability.[1-3]

The concept of 3D echocardiography started in the early 90s. Previously, dynamic cardiac 3D-rendered images were possible using an off-line process, by sequentially acquiring 2D images, outputting these images to disk or CD-ROM, and using a workstation to input the 2D images for Cartesian coordinate conversion. The result was a tedious, time-consuming process. Outside of a research setting, this cumbersome process proved costly in terms of productivity and the ability to provide quality patient care.

While three-dimensional imaging of the heart and its structures is already state of-the-art with other tomographic imaging technologies including radionuclear, magnetic resonance and computed tomography, progress in three-dimensional echocardiography has been rather slow. In its early stages, three-dimensional echocardiography was applied mainly in volume measurement of the left ventricle using static wire frame pictures, which may demonstrate the shape of the ventricular cavity, but does not provide tissue-depicting information. Recently, along with the rapid evolution in computer technology, three-dimensional echocardiography has grown into a well-developed technique able to display dynamic images of the heart that contain tissue information and show the depth of the structures in their realistic forms. These capabilities undoubtedly provide an improved understanding of unpredictable pathomorphology and decrease the variability both in the quality and interpretation of complex pathology among investigators. Advantages of three-dimensional echocardiography are presented in Table 1. In particular, the availability and versatility using the volumetric data set, showing cardiac anatomy and pathology in projections that have not been possible until now, offer significant advantages.

OFF-LINE 3D RECONSTRUCTION

IMAGE ACQUISITION

Currently available methods for data acquisition include:

Linear Scanning

The transducer translates perpendicularly to the imaging plane, linearly over the patient's skin, in discrete, equal steps. This is accomplished by mounting a conventional linear or curved transducer in an assembly housing a motor and drive mechanism. Parallel images are stored and digitally combined to create a third dimension. Linear scanning has been used in conjunction with intravascular ultrasound catheters to create endocardial casts, representations of the inner arterial architecture that are particularly useful in the elucidation of complex vascular lesions.

TABLE 1 Advantages of 3D Echocardiography

I. Valvular heart disease	**Details of advantages**
1. Mitral valve anatomy	Identifies the prolapsing and flail scallops, helps in mitral valve repair
Mitral regurgitation	Direct measurement of effective regurgitant orifice area at the level of vena contracta,
Mitral stenosis	Assessment of the smallest mitral valve orifice and splitting of commissures
2. Aortic valve anatomy	Assessment of bicuspid aortic valve, assessment for aortic valve repair and quantification of aortic stenosis. Direct measurement of ERO in AR
3. Tricuspid valve	Accurate assessment of the tricuspid annulus for surgical decision making processes
II. Assessment of Cardiac Chambers, Volumes and Dyssynchrony	
1. Assessment chamber volume and ejection fraction	Accurate assessment of left ventricular volume and ejection fraction, LV mass comparable to MRI Assessment of left atrial volume Assessment of RV volume and function 3D echo derived LV systolic dyssynchrony index is highly predictive of response to CRT
2. Stress echocardiography	(1) Better visualization of the LV apex, (2) Rapid acquisition of peak stress images, (3) Evaluation of multiple segments from different planes from a single data set
III. Congenital Heart Disease	
	1. Diagnosis, Typing of ASD, PFO during and after device closure 2. Accurate identification of size and site of the ventricular septal defect 3. To obtain en face image of the sub aortic membrane
IV. During Percutaneous interventions and Surgery	
1. During Interventional procedures	1. During ASD device closure 2. During mitral valve clips 3. Transcatheter aortic valve implantations 4. Para valvular regurgitation-device closure 5. Guides atrial septal puncture 6. Guides pulmonary vein ablation for AF
2. Intraoperative 3D echocardiography	1. During mitral valve repair 2. During septal myectomy in patients with hypertrophic cardiomyopathy

Rotational Scanning

A motor rotates the transducer array from 0 to 180° around an axis that is perpendicular to the array. This rotation geometry allows the axis of rotation to be fixed, while the acquired images sweep out, producing a conical imaging volume.

Fan-like or Tilt Scanning

The mechanical assembly tilts the transducer about an axis parallel to the axis of transducer. The process of acquiring 2D images at fixed intervals during the tilt motion or at regular angular intervals results in the computer storage of a set of 2D image planes arranged in a fan-like geometry. This technique allows image acquisition from a small acoustic window. The array is moved from a fixed point in a sweeping motion that spans approximately –60° to +60°, producing a pyramidal image volume.

FREE-HAND SCANNING

Although the mechanical scanning approach to ultrasonography offers speed and accuracy at times the bulkiness and weight of the devices hinder the scan. To overcome this problem many investigators have attempted to develop various free-hand scanning techniques in which the operator can hold the transducer with a position sensor attachment and manipulate it over the anatomy in the usual manner. This technique requires the operator to scan steadily over the precordial surface at a uniform speed. A number of free-hand scanning approaches have been developed that make use of four basic position sensing techniques: acoustic, articulated arm, image correlation methods and magnetic field. In the last one approach, a pulsed magnetic field is used to track the array's position in 3D space. A small magnetic receiver is attached to the transducer housing and a magnetic field transmitter is located close to the patient chest. Because of the magnetic field created around the chest, freehand scanning should not be used if the patient's heart rate is pacemaker-dependent.

IMAGE PROCESSING AND ANALYSIS

Off-line 3D reconstruction requires a series of steps including:

CONVERSION

The digital data are stored in their original 2D format and must be converted to a rectangular coordinate system for reconstruction (post-processing).

INTERPOLATION

It consists of assigning pixel intensities to fill in existing gaps. After conversion and interpolation, the pixels are treated as spatially correct 3D image elements known as voxels.

SEGMENTATION

It consists of delineating the ROI that contains the information required for reconstruction. Segmentation allows tissue and blood to be separated and displayed individually.

IMAGE ENHANCEMENT

Because of fuzzy ultrasound images and noise, including artifacts, the manipulation of 3D data sets from a 2D video screen requires graphics enhancements such as histograms and filtering.

VOLUME RECONSTRUCTION

After the 2D images have been acquired and their relative position and orientation determined, the 3D data can be reconstructed. This process refers to the generation of a 3D representation of the anatomy and involves placing each acquired 2D image at its correct relative position to all the other images. The 3D reconstruction process can be implemented using two distinct methods: feature based and voxel based.

REAL-TIME 3D ECHOCARDIOGRAPHY OR LIVE 3D ECHOCARDIOGRAPHY

Live three-dimensional echocardiography is a breakthrough in the field of medical ultrasound. The idea of real-time 3D cardiac sonography is not new. Clinicians have been experimenting with the manipulation of 2D images to come up with 3D images for twenty years. In the past, dynamic cardiac 3D rendered images were possible by sequentially acquiring 2D images and then using a workstation to input 2D images for Cartesian coordinate conversion and volume rendering. Outside research settings, this time-consuming process proved cumbersome and was simply impractical. Real-time volumetric 3D echocardiography employs a matrix array that generates a pyramidal burst of ultrasound. It requires very rapid beam formation and data processing, only possible with parallel-processing system, which permits the reception of 16 signals in return for each transmitted impulse. The beam is steered in both elevational and azimuthal directions.

MATRIX TRANSDUCER

The first matrix array transducers for live 3D echocardiography were developed by Duke University, but the currently available probes and the system are commercially manufactured by Philips Corporation (Bothell, WA, USA). Laser is used to cut the piezoelectric crystal into many equal-sized minute square elements, forming an element matrix. The most commonly used transducer at present consists of more than 3600 (60_60) to 6400 (80_80) elements with operating frequencies ranging between 2 and 4 MHz. These elements are housed in the tip of the transducer so that they can be in close contact with the surface of the body for easy transmission and reception of ultrasound pulses.

STEERING 3D SOUND BEAM BY PHASED ARRAY

The matrix transducer generates ultrasonic beams in a phased array manner. The computer controls emissions in multiple directions and controls the timing of element firing. Each fired element produces an ultrasonic wave beam, and following Huygens principle, the wave beams combine to form a wave front. If all of the elements are fired simultaneously, the direction of the wave front will be perpendicular to the surface of the probe. By delaying the firing time of some elements, ultrasonic wave beams are created in different phases. Thus, the direction of the wave front can be altered by adjusting this delay time. So, although the probe is maintained in a stable orientation, the ultrasonic beam can change direction and reach any targeted area. The ultrasonic beam goes along the predetermined X-axis and produces a scanning line from near to far. The scanning line performs azimuth steering along Y-axis in the phased array manner and produces a 2D sector image. The 2D sector image then performs elevation steering along Z-axis and finally produces the pyramidal 3D image data set.

BOTTLENECK OF REAL-TIME 3D ULTRASOUND

With the matrix transducer, the theory of rapidly scanning and obtaining a pyramidal 3D dataset was established. The remaining problem was how to control the procedure to image in real time and to emit pulses with a computer. For example, suppose the size of the pyramidal 3-D image dataset is 60° _ 30° and one scanning line in every 1" of the 60° 2D sector image is generated by azimuth steering along Y-axis. Then, at every 1" in the 30° elevation steering along Z-axis, there will be one frame of 2D sector image as well, so 60 Y-axis sections by 30 Z-axis sections makes 1800 scanning lines for one pyramidal 3D image dataset. According to a study by Roget in 1824, the persistence of human vision is about 1/24 of a second. Therefore, in order to achieve live 3-D images, we must obtain at least 24 pyramidal 3-D image datasets per second. To observe the stereo continuous movement of heart structures, the scanning lines generated by the live 3D system every second would be the scanning lines (1,800) of one pyramidal 3D data set multiplied by 24 (frame rate). Then, 43,200 scanning lines are needed in 1 second, the minimal pulse repetition frequency is 43.2 KHz and, subsequently, the maximal interval between the two consecutive pulses is only 23.1 _s. Given that the average propagation speed of ultrasound is about 1500 m/sec in soft tissues, these pulses could only travel a distance of 3.47 cm in that time for an imaging distance of only 1.73 cm. Such a small depth is not adequate for clinical imaging, which usually requires a depth of over 10 cm.

SOLUTION TO BOTTLENECK PROBLEM

In order to resolve this difficulty, the researchers at Duke University (Durham, NC) and Philips Corporation (Bothell, WA) developed a new microelectronic pulse transmitting-receiving technique, which is characterized by16:1 parallel processing to scan a pyramidal volume instead of the usual 1:1. This technology allowed many ultrasonic scanning beams to be emitted at the same time. As the pulse repetition frequency increases, the interval of the pulses increases 16 times with 16:1 parallel processing, which also increases the depth of ultrasound transmission through body tissues. By this approach, when the pulse repetition frequency is 43.2 KHz, the pulse interval is increased 16 times from 23.1 to 370 s, and the imaging depth from 1.73 cm to 27.7 cm without depth ambiguity.

BIPLANE MODE

Another benefit of the xMATRIX transducer technology is the possibility to display two orthogonal images in real time.

CLINICAL APPLICATIONS

Three-dimensional echocardiography has produced promising results from both experimental and clinical studies in the past two and half decades. Favorable experience has been gained in its clinical applications with both transthoracic and transesophageal image data acquisition.

VOLUME QUANTIFICATION

Echocardiography is a widely available clinical method, which consents to measure diastolic and systolic volumes and derived parameters, such as ejection fraction. Precision and accuracy of echocardiographic measurements is typically compromised by user subjectivity and geometrical assumption about left ventricular shape. The rationale behind the accuracy and reproducibility of volume measurement with three-dimensional echocardiography in comparison with any two-dimensional method is that the three-dimensional approach obviates any geometric assumptions of the shape of the measured object. Good correlations with angiography, magnetic resonance imaging and anatomical measurements (*in vitro*) have been reported. At present, ventricular volumes are calculated by manual endocardial tracing of sequential short-axis views derived by parallel slicing through three-dimensional data set at prescribed thickness intervals at either end-systole or end-diastole. Volume quantification is achieved by the summation of the voxels included in the traced area with the subsequent summing of the subvolumes of each slice with known slice thickness. Stroke volume and ejection fraction of a given chamber can be derived from its end-systolic and end-diastolic volumes.

VALVULAR HEART DISEASE

Both qualitative and quantitative evaluation of valvular heart disease can be improved by three-dimensional echocardiography. Any plane and paraplane analysis of the stenotic valve helps to find the smallest orifice area for accurate planimetry. Mitral valve prolapse is visualized as a bulging or protrusion on the atrial side together with its exact location and extension, allowing the surgeon to better plan the repair procedures. Three-dimensional echocardiography has been shown to be highly accurate for identifying the flail scallop. Three-dimensional echocardiography may further help in the quantitative evaluation of valvular abnormalities by improved analysis of the proximal flow convergence. Research is currently directed towards reconstruction of regurgitant jets showing the site of origin, trajectory and both the geometric distribution and morphology of the jet.

CONGENITAL HEART DISEASE

Three-dimensional echocardiography has been proven valuable in congenital heart disease for better evaluation of morphologic abnormalities and understanding of complex spatial relationships. Computer reconstruction of enface views of an atrial or ventricular septal defect, visualized from its right or left side, not only provides a surgeon's view of the defect before the heart is open but also enables accurate measurement of the dimensions of the defect and of the tissues surrounding the defect, the latter being crucial for planning closed-chest closure of the defect using a transcatheter closing device.

CORONARY ARTERY DISEASE

Coronary heart disease is one of the most commonly encountered diseases for the cardiologist. Three-dimensional echocardiography has shown its potential in accurate evaluation of volumes and function of the ventricles, in the analysis and quantitative measurements of regional wall motion abnormalities and myocardial perfusion territories using contrast agents Initial experience indicates that three-dimensional visualization of the proximal segments of the coronary arteries is possible.

CARDIOMYOPATHY

High-resolution Live 3D Echo allows a comprehensive analysis of LV wall motion before and during CRT and in contrast to conventional 2D Echo—the comparison of all LV segments. Live 3D Echo used in conjunction with a quantitative contour tracing algorithm allows comparison of asynchronism between all segments, while providing intuitive display of ventricular synchronicity. In addition it allows clinicians to obtain quantifiable data, it may provide a good prediction of CRT responders, can aid in optimizing pacemaker settings and Live 3D Echo enables rapid image acquisition.

CARDIAC MASSES

Three-dimensional echocardiography has been used in almost all aspects of cardiac disorders and various benefits have been derived. Evaluation of intracardiac or intravascular masses including vegetations, tumors, thrombi or plaques is facilitated both qualitatively (by three dimensional display of their site, size, attachment and mobility) and quantitatively (by accurate measurement of their dimensions and volumes).

AORTIC DISEASES

Aortic diseases such as dilation, aneurysm, dissection or coarctation with three-dimensional echocardiography and incremental information was obtained.

PLANNING CARDIAC SURGERY

Live 3D Echo improves spatial orientation and accesses critical views of the heart, aiding surgeons in the observation and quantification of size, shape and volume of the heart. One of the most important methods in assessing heart function is measuring left ventricular volumes during the cardiac cycle. Since accuracy is critical in assessing and quantifying the condition of the heart, Live 3D Echo is a much better option than other imaging methods as it enables clinicians to make measurements using an offline software tool without making geometric assumptions, which can prove costly. In addition to preoperative planning, Live 3D Echo is important in evaluating and monitoring surgical outcomes by performing real-time assessments of understanding will help improve patient throughput, training, patient communication and marketing.

Live 3D Echo contributes to improved clinical efficiencies with the potential to speed up diagnostic and interventional procedural time. The ability to obtain more complete diagnostic information decreases time spent studying clinical information and provides a higher degree of confidence in those results. The mobility of the ultrasound equipment also provides advantages. Ultrasound is simple and easily performed at the patient's bedside, providing real time results, thereby enhancing patient throughput and reducing wait times.

TRAINING AND PATIENT EDUCATION

Training is another area of operations that will realize significant improvements and cost savings. Two-dimensional cardiac ultrasound required a steep learning curve, which made training time consuming and expensive, since it required visualizing the heart three-dimensionally in 2D pieces in order to understand the results. Live 3D Echo provides the ability to quickly view the heart as it really appears, instantaneously in 3D, which sharply reduces this learning curve, reduces training costs and time spent getting clinicians up to speed.

Two-dimensional ultrasound makes little sense to patients wanting to know and understand their own healthcare. The ability to show patients easily understandable 3D images of their hearts will make it easier for clinicians to explain these images to patients. This not only speeds time clinicians spend with patients but also gives patients a higher level of comfort in what they are being told as they will better understand what their healthcare provider is showing them.

CONCLUSION

Live 3D Echo is a significant new advancement in ultrasound that is changing the way in which cardiology is practiced from the clinic all the way to the operating room. As a result, live 3D Echo is advancing the level of care provided to patients, which will ultimately have a positive impact on an institution's bottom line.

REFERENCES

1. Lang RM, Badano LP, Wendy Tsang, et al. EAE/ASE Recommendations for image acquisition and display using Three-dimensional echocardiography J Am Soc Echocardiogr 2012;25:3-46.
2. Judy Hung, Lang RM, Frank Flachskampf, et al. 3D Echocardiography : A review of the current status and future directions J Am Soc Echocardiogr 2007;20:213-33.
3. Alexandra Gonçalves, José Luis Zamorano. Valve Anatomy and function with transthoracic three-dimensional echocardiography : advantages and limitations of instantaneous full volume color Doppler imaging. Ther Adv Cardiovasc Dis 2010;4:385.

CHAPTER 2

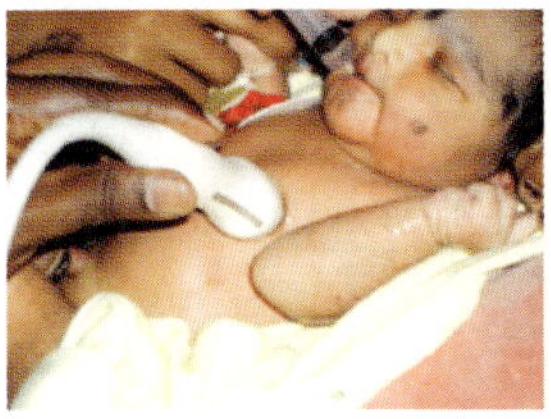

How to Perform the 3D Echocardiography

V Amuthan

INTRODUCTION

Echocardiography has been the marvel of 20th century. This ultrasound technique since its inception from the days of Elder, has revolutionalized the diagnosis and treatment in the management of cardiac patients. From the days of single crystal probe to M Mode, 2D, Color flow mapping, the advancement has reached the stage of 3Dimentional Echocardiogram. The cumbersome big mechanical probes are now replaced with smaller X Matrix probes which can acquire images from a single cardiac cycle.[1-3] Let us see step by step approach to 3D Echocardiogram and Real time 3D transesophageal echocardiogram at the end of this chapter (Tables 1 and 2).

TECHNICAL DEVELOPMENT OF 3D ECHOCARDIOGRAPHY TO DATE

This imaging procedure has been developed in several steps since the initial development of 3D echocardiography ("Echo-CT")[4] in the late 1980s. The broadest use of data acquisition initially involved the rotation procedure on the basis of commercial multiplane TEE-transducers. Later, transthoracic data acquisition with the rotation procedure or the freehand technique were also realized. The limited image resolution of these procedures have been clearly improved by recent developments. The decisive disadvantage of these procedures, however, remains that data acquisition and presentation are not done in real-time. The introduction of the first phased-array real-time volumetric 3D imaging system (Duke University, Durham, North Carolina) enabled transthoracic real-time acquisition of 3D echocardiographic data sets.[5] A breakthrough in the area of transthoracic real-time 3D echocardiography was achieved with the so-called "Live-3D" (Sonos 7500, Philips, Andover, Massachusetts). In addition to transthoracic real-time acquisition, simultaneous presentation of perspective images became possible; the spatial image resolution was considerably improved.

THE PROCEDURE OF 3D ECHOCARDIOGRAPHY

The technological advances have made it possible for the three dimensional echocardiography from a single crystal A-mode to two dimensional B-mode with 2D Phased-array transducer to the 3D Matrix-array (Figure 1A). The 3D Matrix-array transducer acquires a pyramidal cone of data set (Figure 1B). The transducers are slightly larger than the 2D Phased-array transducers (Figure 2A). The performance of the 3D Echocardiogram has the same methodology of standard two dimensional echocardiography.[6-8] The image data set is essentially acquired from the same Para-sternal and apical windows. More commonly the apical window is chosen (Figure 2B). One standard requirement for the aquicision of three dimensional echocardiography is the connection of standard ECG. Another important factor to be kept in mind is the aquicision of optimized two dimensional images. These images can be viewed in three different formats.[9-23]

1. **Live 3D (Narrow Angle):** A narrow angle slice of data set is acquired in real time and can be moved with side to side or above downward orientation (Figures 3A to C).
2. **X Plane View:** Simultaneously orthogonally two opposite planes of two dimensional echocardiograms can be viewed (Figures 4A and B).
3. **Full Volume (Figures 5 and 7):** A full volume of cone of data set is acquired. In the initial versions of the equipments, five cardiac cycles were used for this features. In more recent equipments a single cardiac cycle is used.

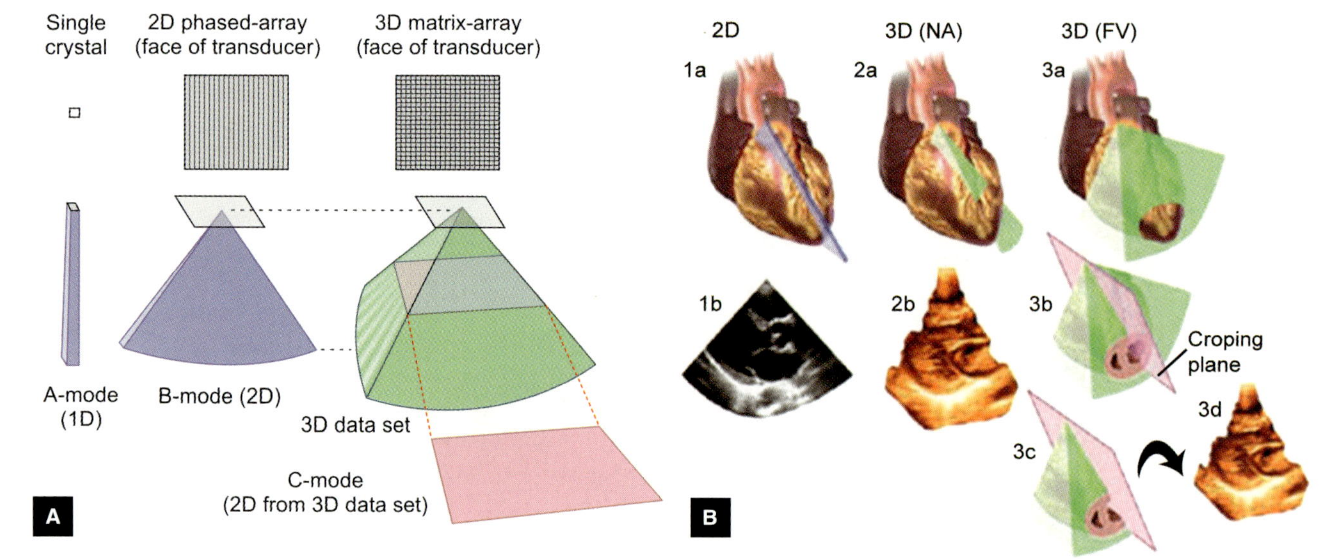

Figures 1A and B: Figure Adapted from Houck RC, Cooke. JE and Gill. EA, AJR 2006; 187:1092–1106 (A) The transition from single crystal A-mode to 2D Phased array transducer and the 3D Matrix array transducer where a larger pyramid of data set is acquired; (B) Comparing the imaging plane in 2D Long axis view 1a and 1b to the Live 3D Narrow angle or thin slice cut – 2a and 2b, with 3D Full volume or thick slice cut 3a and 3b. The Cropping plane can be in the Long axis plane or in the transverse (short axis plane) Full volume is acquired from total of four cardiac cycles. Each individual cardiac cycle contributes one fourth of thickness of entire data set as illustrated with individual colors. Cardiac gating is required to meld four cardiac cycles into one. The modern X5-1 Matrix transducer acquires a full volume in one cardiac cycle

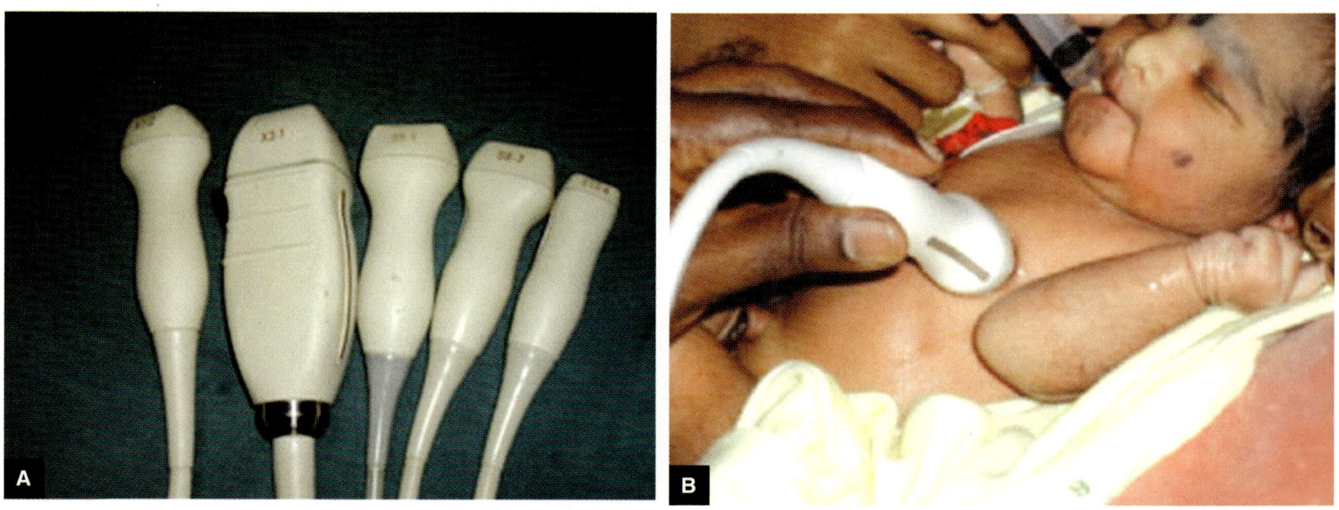

Figures 2A and B: (A) The comparison of the size of 3D Matrix transducers X7-2 (Pediatric), X3-1 (Adult 0, and the routine Phased array 2 D transducers S51, S8-3 and S12-4; (B) Acquisition of the Full Volume 3D image from apical plane in a baby with X7-2

4. **3D Color Full volume:** In this mode, the Color flow mapping can be done within the three-dimensionally acquired image. The advantages of the 3D color full volume acquisition is the ease of identification of the area of vena contracta in regurgitant lesions and to identify the site of regurgitation in differentiation of valvular and para-valvular leaks.[24-27] Table 1 and 2 give the tips and tricks to obtain good 3D transthoracic and transesophageal echocardiographic images.

TOOLS FOR 3D ECHOCARDIOGRAPHY—COLOR CODING

In the full volume three-dimensional viewing, after acquisition, the pyramidal dataset is displayed within a cube for reference. Color coding is used for the cube: Green for Coronal plane from anterior to posterior, Blue for Cranio Caudal and red for Sagital Plane—from left to right and so on. Further Max and Min are used for operation from

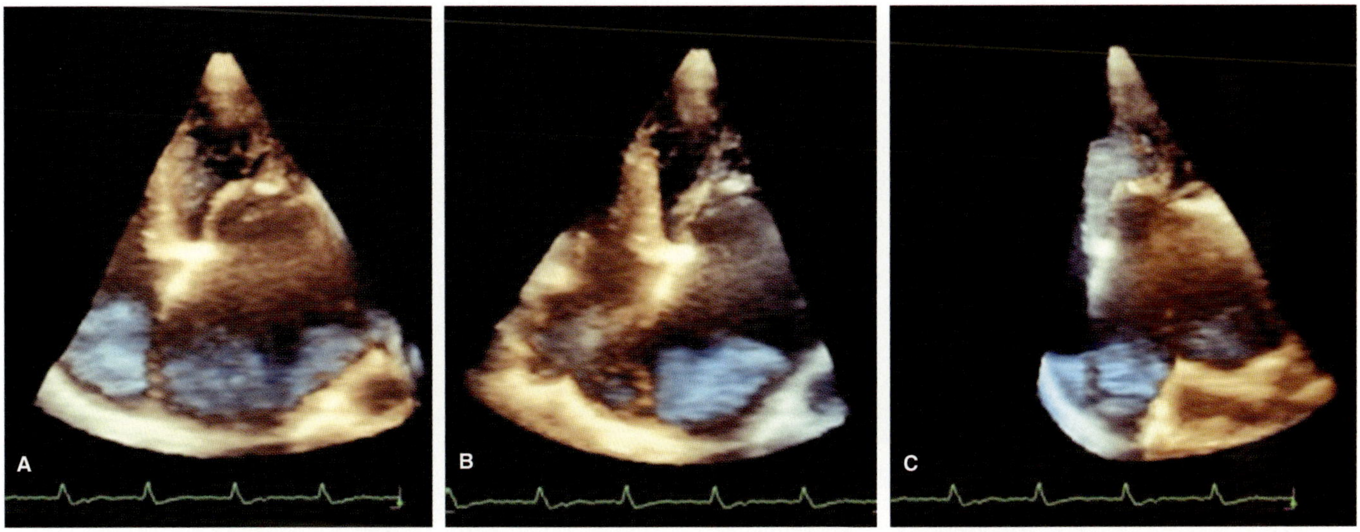

Figures 3A to C: **Live 3D** – Narrow angle slice Examination similar to 2D, with the additional modes of rotation which is possible in all planes—side to side or from above downwards and below upwards

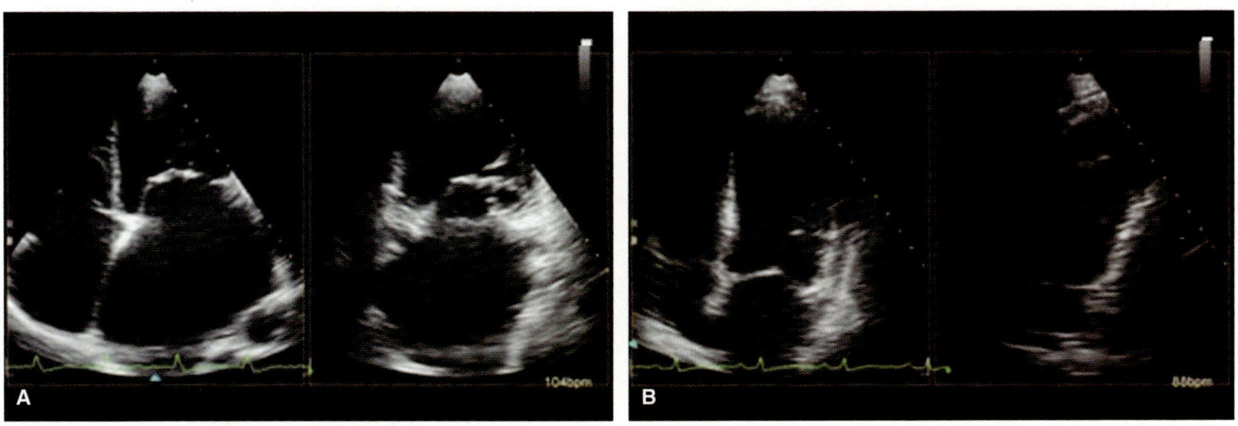

Figures 4 A and B: Examination in X Plane where simultaneous viewing of the 2 dimensional images from two orthogonally opposite planes is possible. By moving the cursor we can cut in different planes either on the centre (Figure 4A in a patient with mitral stenosis) or on the right side (Figure 4B in a patient with LV apical aneurysm) or on the left side

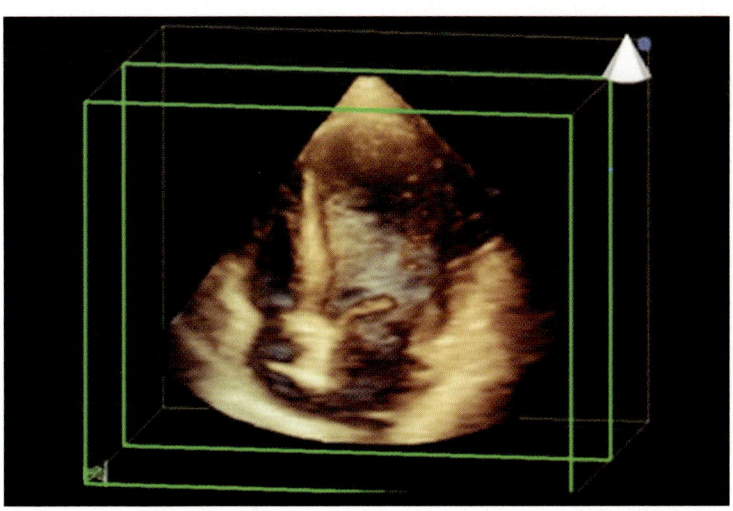

Figure 5: Acquisition of a Full volume 3D cone of image from the apical window and depiction of it with in a cube. After acquisition of Full volume cone of image, automatically, auto cropped image is shown as in this figure. There is color coding for all the different sides: Green for Coronal plane—Anterior to posterior, Blue for Cranio caudal and Red for Sagital plane right to left (Each color is coded as Max and Min for two orthogonally different types of movements). By moving the crop box, the cone of image can be cut at that level

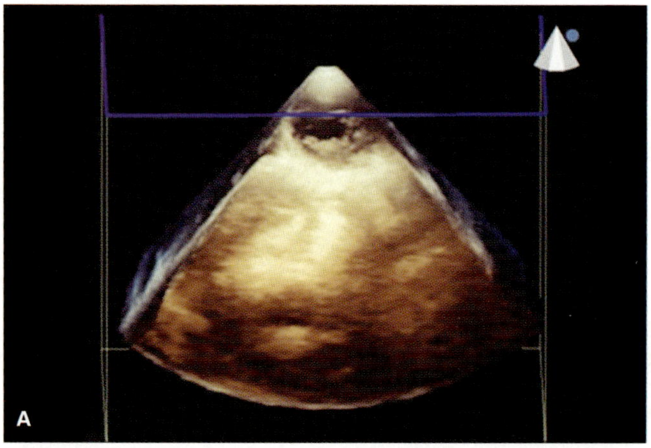

Figure 6A: This auto cropped image can be also seen as a cone of image by using the crop box. Then we can initiate cropping to see the cross sectional images with Blue crop box seen above

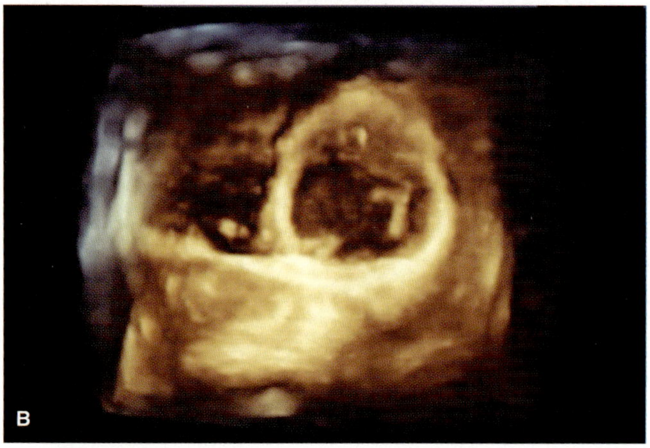

Figure 6B: Cropping from the above – from the apex using the blue crop box. The cross sectional image at the mid Left ventricular level showing the right and left ventricle

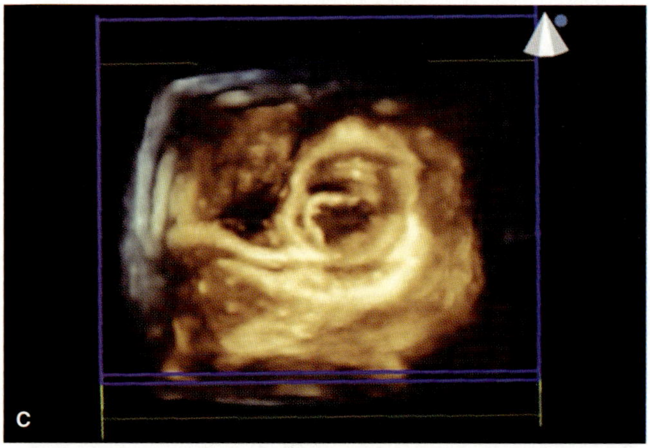

Figure 6C: Cropping to a lower level from the apex: At the level of mitral valve. The anterior and posterior mitral leaflet are seen clearly the scallops from lateral to medial A1, A2 and A3 in the AML and P1, P2 and P3 in the PML

orthogonally opposite sides. For example, Green Max is used to crop from anterior aspect and Green Min is used to crop from posterior aspect.

CROPPING

Cropping is an important tool in three-dimensional echocardiography. The machine after acquisition of the image displays it as an auto cropped image in the Coronal plane. To view the full pyramid, the image can be rotated through 90 degrees and the crop box can be moved in coronal plane. By cropping, the unwanted elements in the images can be removed. Figures 6A to C show how to crop from this pyramidal image and view cross sectional short axis view of mitral valve from below upwards or from above downward from the left atrial side. Oblique crop boxes are also available, which can be used for oblique cropping (Figures 8A and B). See also accompanying video on the CD showing the cropping function.

3D ZOOM VIEWING

By using the zoom tool, a particular area of interest can be enlarged and viewed.

ISCAN

By using this option in the advanced Q Lab software, serial sections at apical, mid LV level and mitral valve level cross sectional short axis cuts can be viewed (Figure 9) similar to Radionucletide studies.

TRANSESOPHAGEAL ECHOCARDIOGRAPHY

Transesophageal echocardiography (TEE) is a necessary tool for cardiologists and cardiac anesthesiologists worldwide. Since the introduction of a TEE probe with a single-crystal M-mode transducer allowing unidimensional imaging, the TEE probe has evolved into a clinically valuable diagnostic tool used for the comprehensive examination of cardiovascular abnormalities. Currently, 3-dimensional (3D) TEE is performed with a multiplane probe using a rotational approach for sequential data acquisition, gated to electrocardiography (ECG) and respiration.[4-7] From these 3D volume datasets, any desired cut plane can be derived and structures of interest rendered. Unfortunately, this technique is limited by lengthy data acquisition, frequent radial artifacts, and the need for offline processing.[8] Consequently,

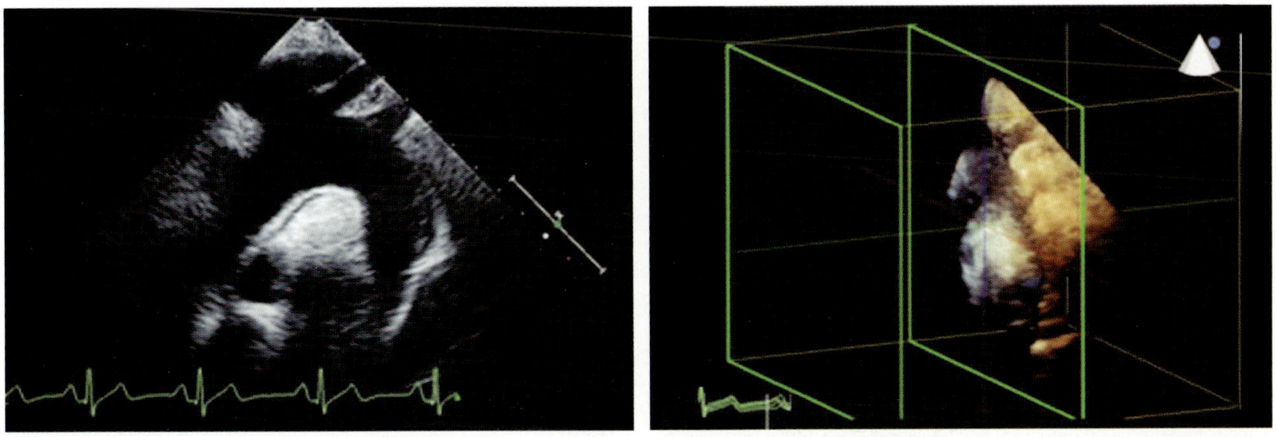

Figure 7: The acquisition of the image of ascending, arch and descending aorta from the supra sternal window is shown as a 2D image on the left and as a Full volume 3D image on the right

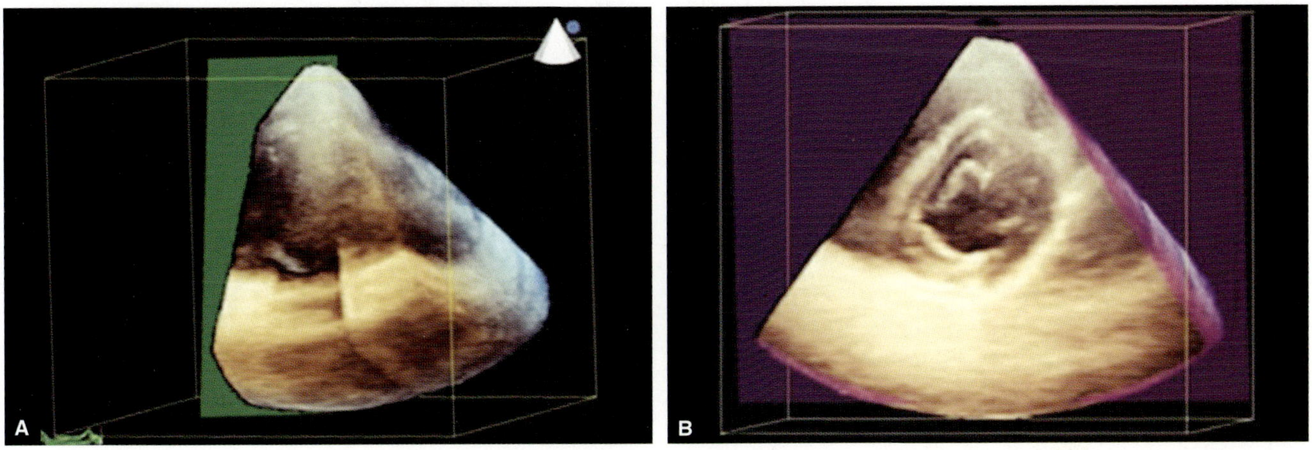

Figures 8A and B: The use of the cropping plane to cut through irregular areas as seen in this figure. After the cut in unusual planes, the image can be rotated and seen from any side

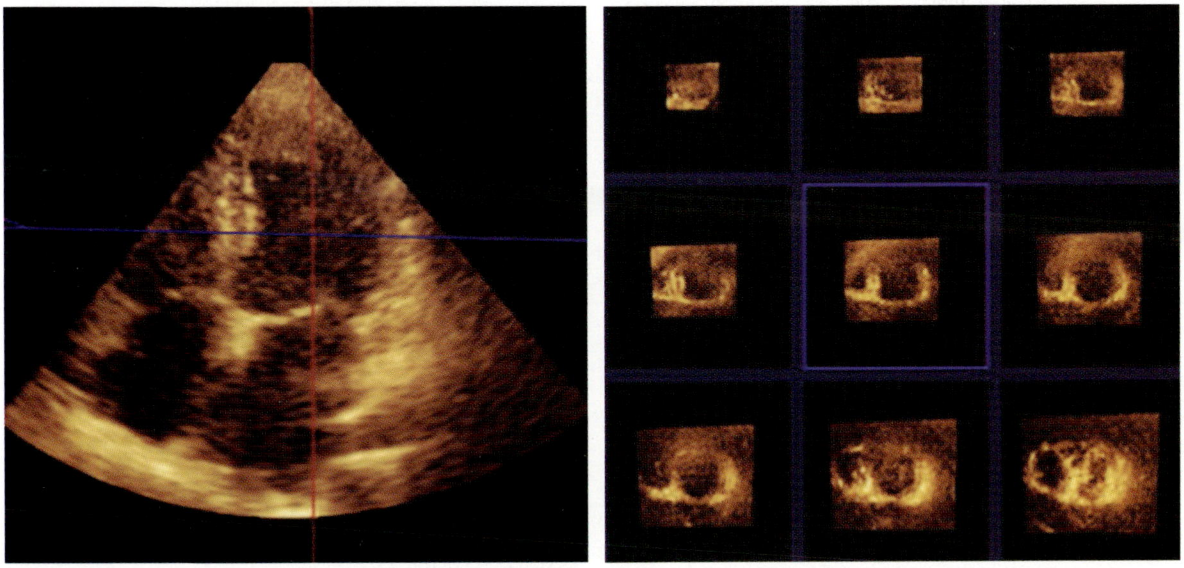

Figure 9: Further analysis is possible with special software in Q Lab. By selecting the advanced version and iScan, cross sectional cuts similar to Radionuclide studies: i.e. apical, Mid LV level and Basal level can be obtained

3D reconstruction TEE has not been embraced routinely in clinical practice and is at this time predominantly used for research. To overcome these limitations, a 3D fully-sampled matrix-array TEE (3D-MTEE) transducer was recently developed to allow real-time acquisition and online display of 3D images. [9-12] This probe combines novel electronic circuitry with miniaturized beam-forming technology in the tip of an otherwise conventional TEE probe.

EQUIPMENT

A typical TEE probe consists of an ultrasound transducer, mounted at the tip of a flexible endoscope. The handle of the probe has two knobs that flex the tip antero posteriorly, or laterally. By advancing, withdrawing, rotating, or flexing the probe, it can be optimally positioned in the patient. There are three main types of transesophageal echocardiographic probes (1) monoplane, (2) biplane, and (3) multiplane (Omniplane). Monoplane probes have a single transducer that images in the transverse plane, at right angles to the probe (0 plane). Biplane probes incorporate a second transducer that images in the longitudinal plane (90 plane). The operator switches back and forth between these orthogonal imaging planes. Multiplane probes have a single transducer that rotates within a housing at the tip of the probe This permits imaging in all planes between 0 and 180, although the transverse and longitudinal planes are used predominantly. Multiplane technology is the current technology used in 2D systems. The core of the Transesophageal real time 3D echocardiography (RT3D-TEE) system is a newly designed semi mechanical Transesophageal probe (Sulzer Innotec, Winterthur, Switzerland). RT3D-TEE probe consists of a cylinder with 24 transducers, which rotates in a protective hull filled with oil. The system uses 5-MHz center frequency; the active aperture of each transducer measures 8 mm. The transducers are arranged in 3 linear groups on 3 sides of the cylinder. The 3 groups are rotated 120° with respect to each other, and in axial direction, they are dislocated relative to each other by 1/3 of the transducer spacing. With this arrangement, 8 planes can be recorded simultaneously in a 120° sector. By completing 1 revolution, 24 planes are recorded. A wedge-like region of 120° and 72 mm in height is acquired in this way with a frame rate corresponding to the number of revolution/s (i.e. 15 to 20 frame/s). The diameter of the round probe tip, including the protective sheath, is 14 mm. The cross-sectional area is thus only slightly larger than the cross-sectional area of commercial 2-dimensional (2D) TEE probes, which have a tip cross-section of about 10 to 14 mm. However, the transducer is nearly 8 cm long, which results in greater rigidity and potentially more difficult intubation of the esophagus. The flexibility of the probe tip is provided by 2 joints to facilitate insertion of the probe in vivo. Thus, the tip of the probe is divided into 3 segments; the middle segment is 4 cm long, and the proximal and distal segments are 2 cm each. Straightening of the probe occurs automatically, owing to the rotational forces, resulting finally in an echo sector with exactly parallel echo planes.

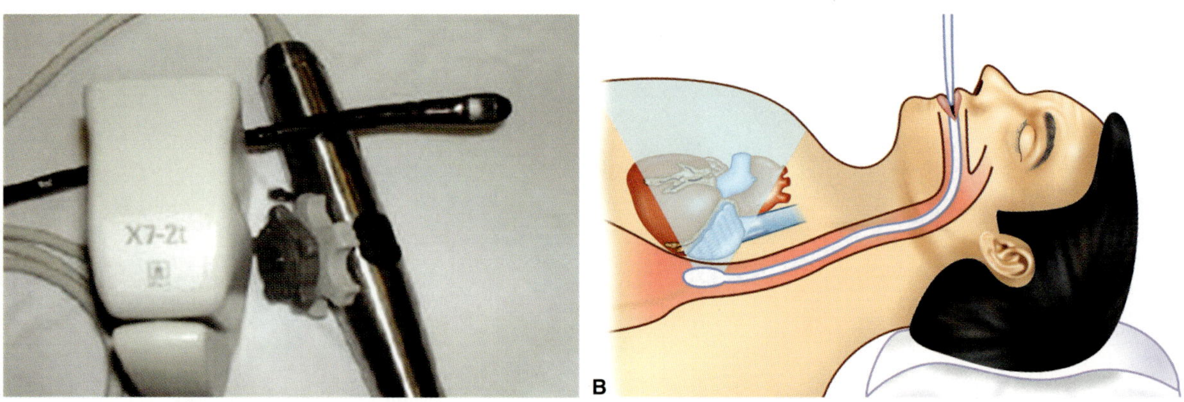

A B

Figures 10A and B: Trans Esophageal Echo and 3D TEE - The 3D TEE probe X7-2t is shown above on the left hand side and on the right hand side, the Trans Esophageal Echocardiography Procedure is shown. The TEE probe is inserted into the Esophagus after light sedation in anxious patients with administration of Lignocaine Viscus with the patient in the left lateral position and through a mouth gag. It is generally safe and in sick patients may require SPO2 monitor. The TEE probe is passed into the stomach at 35 to 40 cm and the Trans Gastric views are obtained. The scope is slowly withdrawn to 30 to 35 cm for lower Esophageal and Mid Esophageal views, then to the Upper Esophageal cuts and finally is rotated to the back to view the descending thoracic aorta

SAFETY CONSIDERATIONS

The torque of the rotating probe is limited to a low level by means of a mechanical system. This should prevent injury to the epithelium, even if the protective sheath should break. Moreover, the sheath is filled with nontoxic oil in case there should be a leak. There is slight warming of the probe of about 2°C due to the rotation. Heating to more than 41°C is prevented by sensors. The probe is rotated by a flexible drive shaft. The ultrasonic signals are supplied via a rotating coupling from an electronic unit, consisting of the transmitter/receiver and digitizer module. The digitized data are then sent to a generic PC, equipped with a powerful graphics engine. The conversion from the raw ultrasonic data stream into a series of stereoscopic images is almost entirely carried out by the graphics engine. An advanced volume-rendering algorithm can generate 20 stereoscopic frames per second. The novel rendering procedure operates in the original cylindrical coordinate system that the data are scanned in.[13]

THE PROCEDURE OF 3D TEE

The 3D TEE probe X7-2t is shown in Figure 10A and the procedure of the transesophageal echocardiography is depicted in Figure 10B. The TEE probe is inserted after a light sedation in anxious patients. Prior to the procedure local anesthesia with Xylocaine-spray is applied to the pharynx. Xylocaine gel is used to lubricate the probe. A mouth gag is used and the probe is advanced into the oral cavity and then into the Esophagus in the left lateral decubitus position. The probe could be introduced without sedation in 2 minutes. The examination generally lasts for a total of about 10 minutes. The procedure is generally safe, and in sick patients may require SPO_2 monitoring. The TEE probe is passed into the stomach at 35 go 40 cm and the Trans Gastric views are obtained. The scope is slowly withdrawn to 30 to 35 cm for lower Esophageal and Mid Esophageal views, then to Upper Esophageal cuts and finally is rotated backwards to view the descending Aorta (Figure 11). Generally a scheme very similar to 2Dimensional Trans Esophageal Echocardiography is followed. However there are very important differences which will be enumerated below. Imaging is performed by using an iE33 ultrasound system (Philips Medical Systems, Andover, Massachusetts) which is equipped with a fully-sampled 3D-MTEE transducer. This transducer uses approximately 3,000 elements, in contrast to the 64 elements currently used in the multiplane TEE probe (i.e. Omni III, Philips Medical Systems).

LIVE 3D

Initially, gain settings are optimized with the narrow-angled acquisition mode (live 3D), which allows real-time 3D imaging without the need for ECG gating. This mode displays a pyramidal volume of approximately 30 to 60°.

THE 3D ZOOM MODE

The Zoom mode displays a smaller, magnified pyramidal volume, is subsequently used to image different cardiac structures, including native valves, Fossa ovalis, and the Left Atrial Appendage.

FULL VOLUME ANALYSIS

In addition, the LV is imaged with the full-volume mode gated to ECG, which acquires 4 narrower wedges of volume over 4 consecutive heart beats, resulting in a wider pyramidal volume (65– 56° up to 102–105°). Images can be also reviewed offline on an workstation with the use of QLAB software (Philips Medical Systems). The high success rate of esophageal intubations with the 3D-MTEE probe is not surprising, considering that the size of the probe

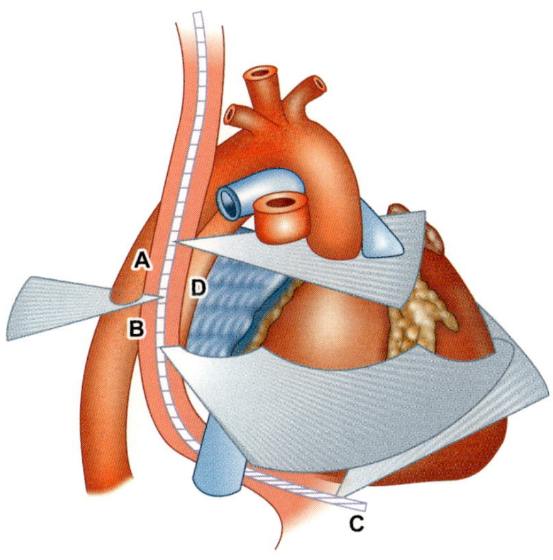

Figure 11: The various levels of cut taken during Trans Esophageal Echocardiography procedure
A: Upper Esophageal cuts
B: Mid and Lower Esophageal cuts
C: Trans Gastric views (35 to 40 cm)
D: Descending Aortic (Posterior) views

TABLE 1 Tips for acquisition an image processing in Transesophageal Echocardiogram

- Optimize 2D image first using 2D Opt, iScan, depth and focus settings
- Go to 3D image
- Check 2D Opt and adjust TGC and overall gain if necessary
- Use 2D reference images if required (under image on left touchscreen)

Using 3D Zoom

- Get desired anatomy in 2D (can use seek angle)
- Optimize 2D image-remember to reduce near—field gain where appropriate
- Press 3D Zoom on right touch screen (RTS)
- Adjust zoom box in preview. Use trackball to adjust size and position in lateral plane (left quad), and use elevation width control on RTS to change size of box in the elevation plane, (Ensure that entire ROI is included in the box without over-sizing) Check image quality adjusting 3 TGC/2D Opt if necessary, then acquire. (Remember to accept volume if accept prior to store is turned on)

Live 3D Acquistion

Using 3D Full Volume

- Ensure good quality ECG trace
- Optimize 2D image as before
- Select full volume (RTS)
- Adjust density to change size of volume, and Full Volume opt to optimize for best frame rate or biggest volume if necessary
- Suspend breath or ventilation
- Acquire
- Autocropped image will be displayed .Check for image quality and ECG triggering, then select accept or reject on LTS as required
- Go back to 2D

Using color 3D Full Volume

Same as 3D full Volume, plus:

- Select color on RTS and optimize-gain, scale, wall filter
- Use trackball to adjust height and position of color box, and use density key to adjust width of color box
- Use Fv Opt key to optimize for best frame rate or biggest volume size if needed
- Suspend breathing or ventilation
- Acquire. Auto cropped image will be displayed. Check for image quality, and accept or reject image.

TABLE 2 Tips for ideal 3D Image acquisition

3D Full volume acquisition

- Optimize your 2D image-iscan, xRes, depth, focus, etc.
- Ensure good quality ECG trace
- Select full volumes on right touch screen (RTS). If you are going to use 3DQA to measure LV volumes, EF and synchronicity ensure you have a four-chamber view in the left-hand sector
- **Get the best image definition** (For LV analysis you can take a foreshortened view or five-chamber view if these give better endocardial definition.) Remember the image on the right is a 90 degree cut to the image on the left
- Ensure the structure of interest is within the bold blue lines and can be seen clearly in both sectors . The "spread" of the bold blue line can be adjusted by using the density control on RTS
- Use density control in conjunction with FV Opt key on RTS if necessary to optimize acquisition for highest frame rate (Frame Rate) or largest volume (Vol size)
- Press acquire, keeping still and using breath hold techniques if necessary
- Autocropped image will be displayed after acquisition is complete. Check image quality and ECG triggering, and press accept or reject on LTS as required

Contd...

Contd...

Live 3D acquisition

- Optimize your 2D image as before. Then select Live 3D
- Default vision map H tags a blue color onto the furthest structure from the eye as the volume is moved to reduce need for cropping and help depth perception

Remember:

- It may be necessary to adjust transducer position slightly for best window
- It may be necessary to adjust your 3D gain by a few percentage points but be cautious–gain too low will give you black holes where data should be, and gain too high will give a cloudy image. Note that some black holes in your data may be "natural", e.g. a structure may be too large for the Live 3D data volume and naturally fall out of its limits
- Move the data volume using the trackball
- Line density defaults to medium by high can be selected for a smaller volume with higher line density. Elevation defaults to back (3D volume extends back from intial 2D scanning plane), but front or center can be selected on RTS to alter elevation position of volume. Lateral position of volume can be moved using control on RTS

tip is similar to the existing TEE probe (Omni III). The 3D-MTEE transducer generally provided superb 3D visualization quality of posterior cardiovascular structures and helps to identify unique spatial relationships between structures that were not previously observed with either currently available real-time transthoracic or reconstructed 3D TEE imaging technology.

TRANS GASTRIC VIEWS

Transesophageal electrocardiography (TEE) examination usually starts with passage of the TEE probe into the 35 to 40 cm position and obtaining the Trans Gastric views first. At this position, with Zero degree angulations, a good cross sectional view of left ventricle is obtained. At this level, rotating to Ninety degrees brings out the mitral valve in perspective (Figure 12).

LOWER AND MID ESOPHAGEAL VIEWS

By far, these are the most preferred views by the Echocardiographers and a detailed anatomy at 0 degree (Horizontal Plane), 55 Degrees (Bicommissural view), 90 Degrees (Longitudinal plane) and 120 degrees (Long Axis plane) are obtained.

Horizontal plane at this level is an important landmark view to start with, and can be easily obtained (Figure 13A). The entire posterior aspect of Inter atrial septum can be viewed along with atrio ventricular junction and upper third of the inlet portion of the Interventricular septum. The anterior mitral leaflet with predominantly the A2 Scallop can be seen along with small portion of A3 and A1 and P1 portion of the posterior mitral leaflet can be viewed.

Bicommissural view: Rotating to 55 degrees at this level brings out the panoramic Bicommissural view. Viewing anteriorly, the A1, A2 and A3 scallops of the Anterior mitral leaflet can be seen and viewing posteriorly brings out the P1, P2 and P3 of the Posterior mitral leaflets (Figure 13B). Unlike the 2 D TEE, the 3 D TEE in Live mode (Narrow angle) brings out the scallops beautifully. Any Scallop prolapse can be obtained in this view. Zooming at this level and getting a Full volume trace at this level can be used to study the mitral valve in various anatomic planes especially to obtain the surgeons view (Figure 15). The surgeons view of mitral valve, (Mitral valve as viewed from left atrial side entirely) is also used during interventions of mitral valve especially during Percutaneous Trans Mitral Commisurotomy and mitral valve clippings for mitral valve regurgitation.

Longitudinal plane: 90 degrees angulations at this level is important to identify the most important inferior vena caval rim of the interventricular septum and the superior vena caval rim (Figure 13C).

Long Axis plane: 120 degrees angulations are used to have the Bicameral view of both left and right atria. Color Flow of the Mitral Forward flow and the mitral regurgitation jets can be well obtained in this view. 3D Color Flow acquisition is best done in this view (Figure 13D). A slight tilt at this level also brings the view of the Left atrial Appendage and Appendage clots (Figure 14).

UPPER ESOPHAGEAL VIEWS

At 25 to 30 cms, the Aortic valve and its leaflets can be viewed beautifully (Figure 16). Turning the probe

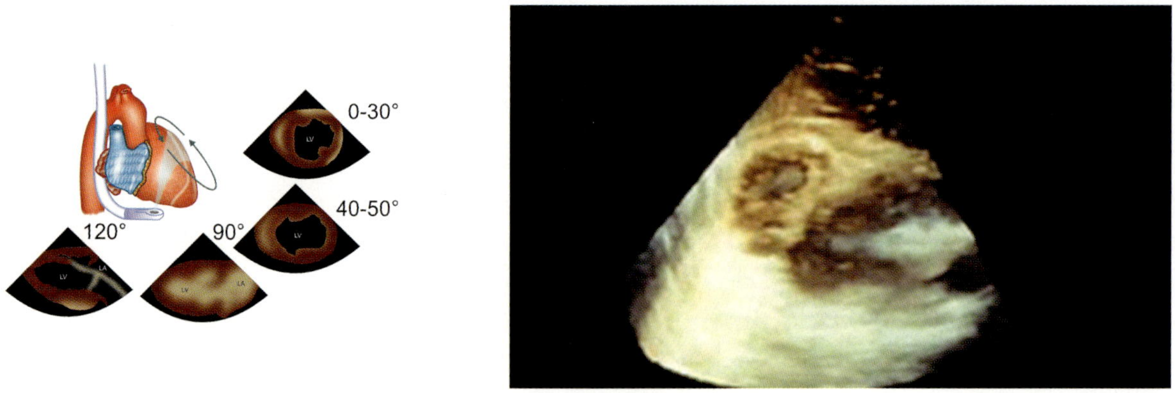

Figure 12: **Trans Gastric views at 35 to 40 cm** with the 3D TEE probe at Zero degree depicting the Left ventricle at the Mid LV level

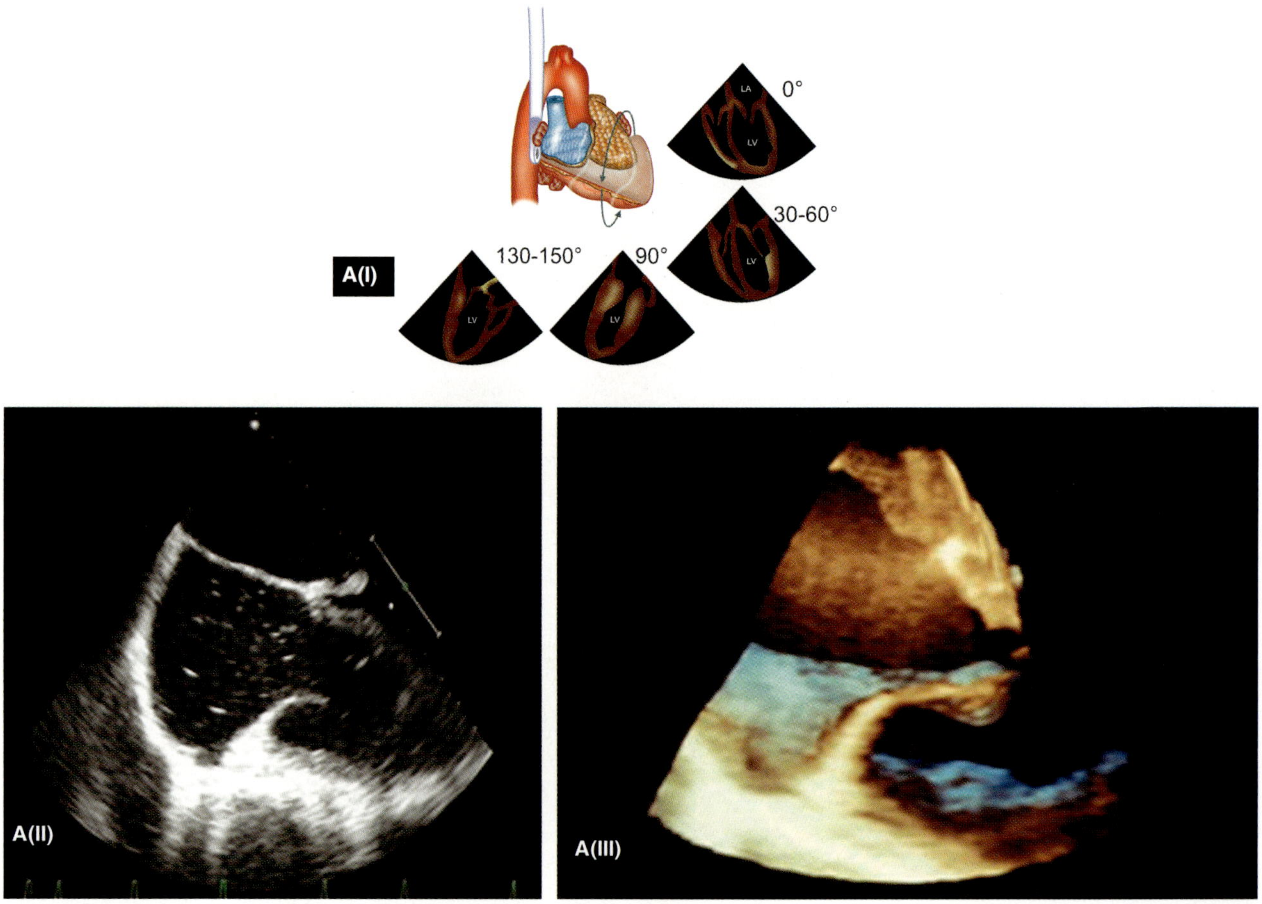

Figure 13 A: **Lower and Mid Esophageal views 30 to 35 cm. A. Horizontal plane:** The Zero degree at this level depicts the inter atrial septum just below the left atrium. The mitral and superior attachments of the inter atrial septum can be well seen and below that the right atrium can be visualized. The mitral and tricuspid attachments and the atrio-ventricular junction can be well made out. It is the usual custom of the Echocardiographers performing TEE, to start from this familiar view as this view is similar to the subcostal four chamber viewing of the heart. The left hand panel depicts the 2D TEE and the right hand panel depicts the Live 3D (Narrow slice) mode. Turning to Full volume trace at this level can be used to bring out the enface view of the atrial septal defect.

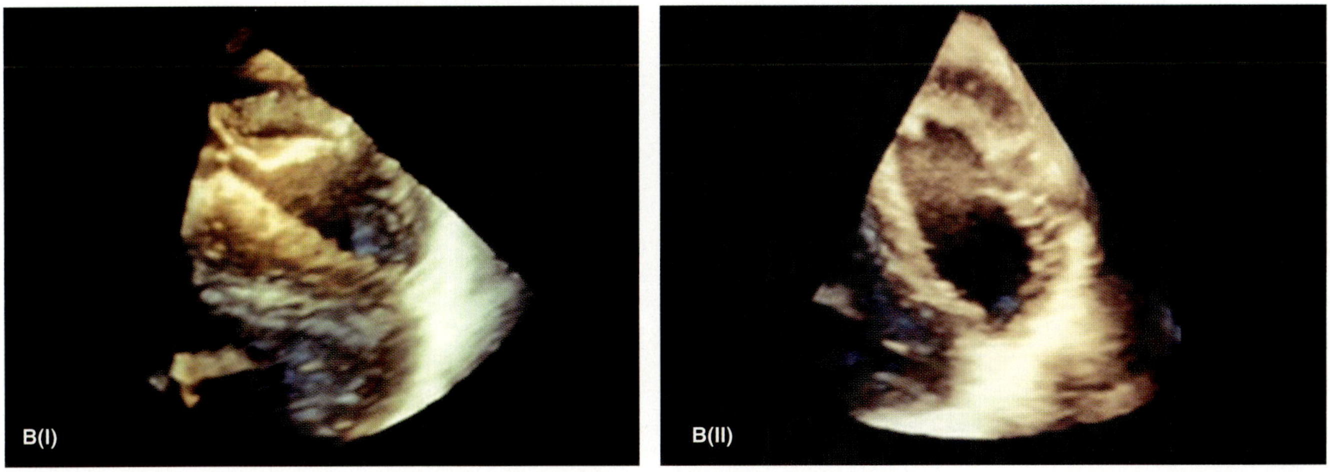

Figure 13 B: **Bicommissural view:** Turning to 55 degrees brings out the bicommissural view of the mitral valve where the cut is made at the level of the medial and lateral commissures and both the leaflets can be seen. Viewing anteriorly at this level, the A1,A2 and A3 scallops of AML from lateral to medial can be seen and viewing posteriorly, the P1,P2 and P3 of PML can be seen

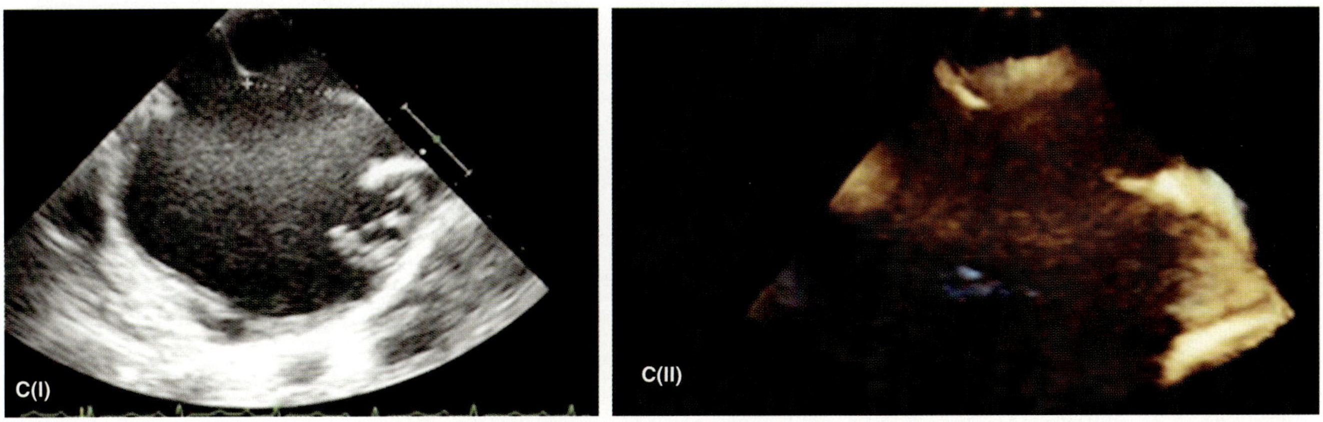

Figure 13 C: **Longitudinal plane or 90 Degrees cut:** In the 90 degrees cut at this level, we can see the inter atrial septum with its superior venae caval and inferior venae caval ends. In patients with atrial septal defect, this view is important to view the SVC and IVC rims to decide about the device closure

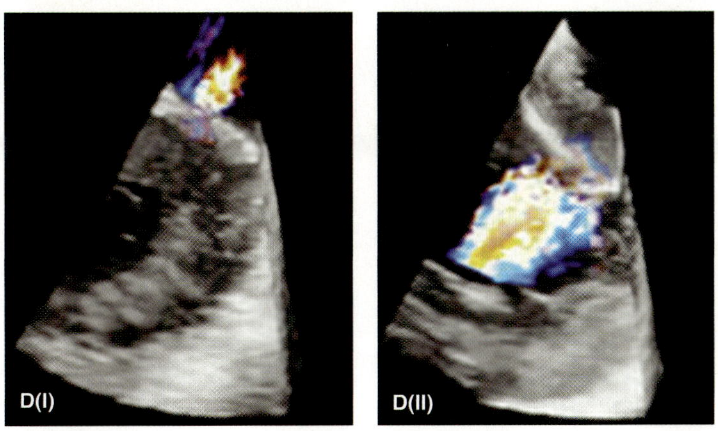

Figure 13 D: **Long Axis Plane or 120 Degrees plane:** This plane corresponds to the trans thoracic parasternal long axis plane. At this level viewing of the Color flow across the mitral valve is possible. In the bottom panel, on the left hand side is the mitral regurgitation jet into left atrium is seen in the 3D TEE Color flow cone. The venae contractae can be accurately visualised and the mitral regurgitation quantified. On the right hand side panel, the mitral stenosis jet can be seen

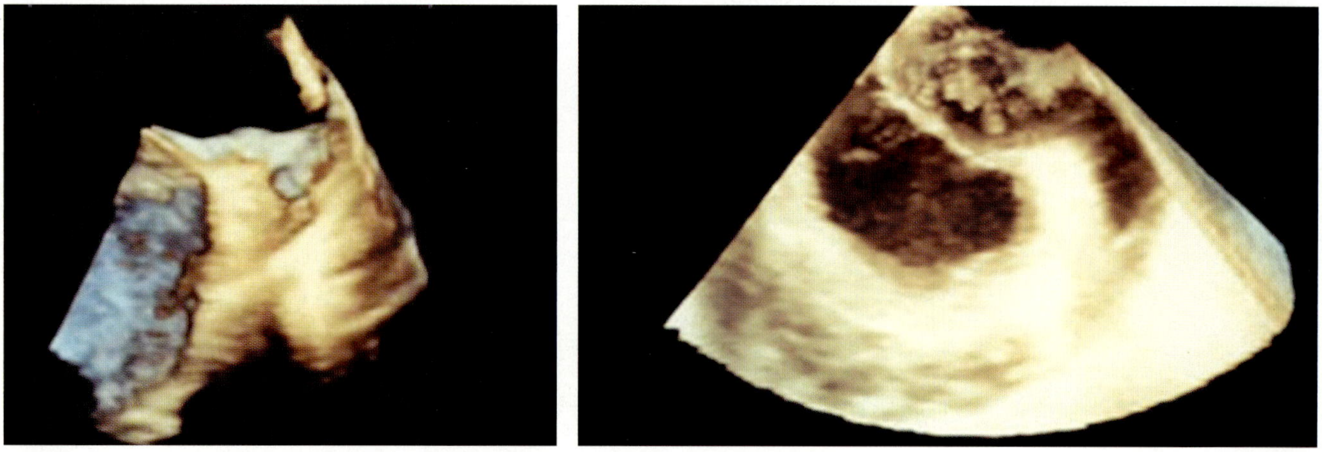

Figure 14: Viewing of the left atrial appendage : Tilting the transducer towards the left atrium we can see the left atrial appendage and the presence of Left atrial appendage clots can be viewed at this level. Left atrial appendage can also be seen in the short axis view at 45 degrees which is shown on the right hand panel

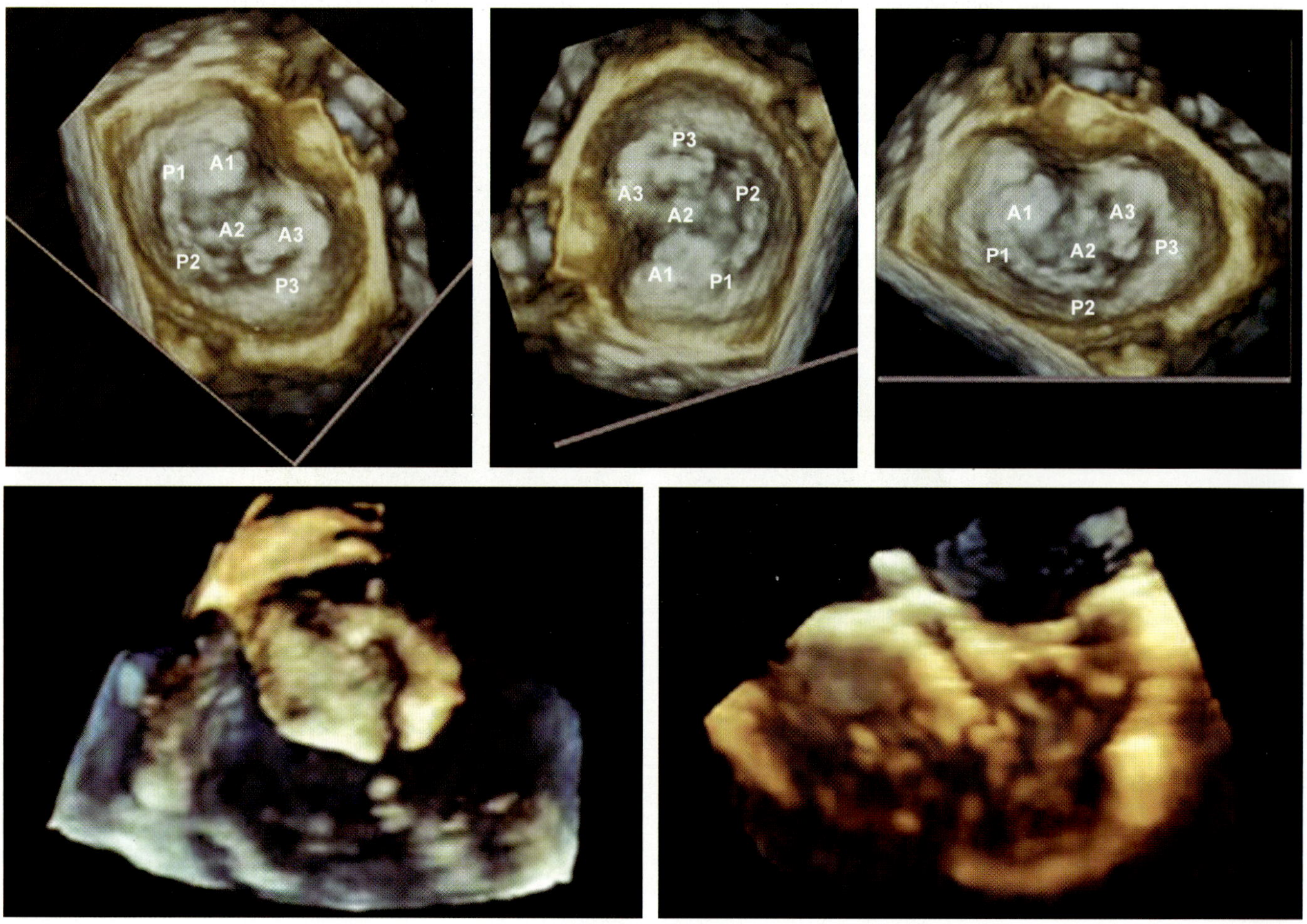

Contd...

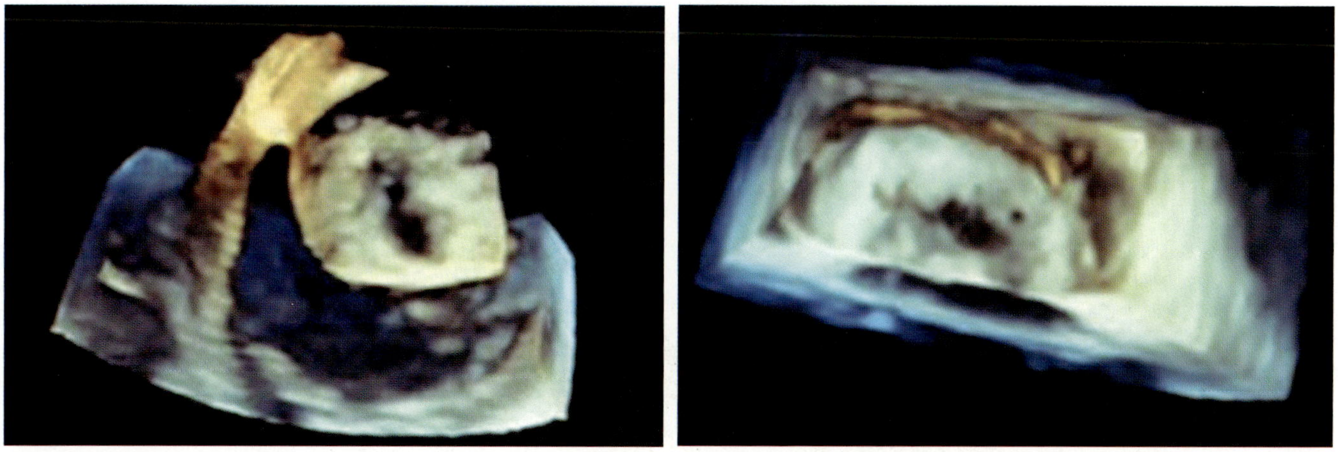

Figure 15: **Viewing of the mitral valve :** The viewing of mitral valve is an important feather in the cap of 3D echocardiography. The mitral valve is a complex structure and can be viewed with ease by echocardiography. The bottom panel A shows anatomical view of the mitral valve which is very difficult to obtain. The panel B shows the trans gastric short axis view obtained after careful maneuvering which is practically difficult. The panel C shows the Surgeons view, which is obtained from the left atrial side in the bicommissural plane, i.e. at 55 degree plane. Panel D shows the mitral valve in the Horizontal plane as viewed from left atrium. Panel E shows the mitral valve as viewed from left ventricle in 3D TEE and Panel F shows the mitral valve as viewed in 40 degrees – 3D TEE short axis plane from left atrial side and Panel G shows the typical Surgeons view of the mitral valve obtained at 55 degrees from left atrial side

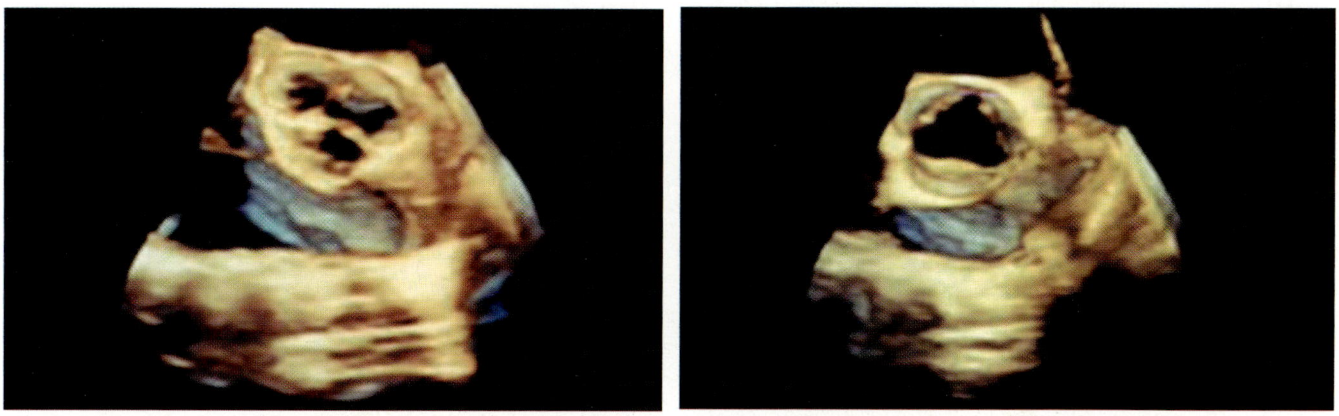

Figure 16: **Upper Esophageal views 25 to 30 cm:** These views are best suited to view the aortic valve with ease bottom panel on the left depicts the trileaflet aortic valve which is a normal valve during diastole and the panel on the right depicts it during systole

posteriorly at this point can be used to view the descending thoracic aorta—especially to view the Aortic Dissection and Coarctation of Aorta.

3D TEE VIEWING OF THE INTER ATRIAL SEPTUM AND ASD

After obtaining a good 2D TEE image in the horizontal 0 degree plane, region of interest is selected by using the X plane imaging in the orthogonally opposite planes to select the potential are of atrial septal defect.[28-34] Then 3D Zoom is selected to have a good view of inter atrial septum. At this point Saric et al have used the **TUPLE Maneuver** (Tilt up and left rotation).[35]

TUPLE MANEUVER I

The initial 3D image of the inter atrial septum seen in Figure 17A is first tilted up along its horizontal axis to reveal an en face view of the inter atrial septum from the right atrial perspective. The superior portion of the inter atrial septum is now on the top of the screen and the anterior portion on the right side of the screen (Figure 17B).

TUPLE MANEUVER II

In the next step, the image of the inter atrial septum is tilted to the left around the vertical axis by approximately 180 degrees until the en face view of the inter atrial septum from the left atrial perspective is obtained. In this view, the superior rim of the inter atrial septum remains at the top of the screen; the anterior (aortic) rim is now on the left side and the ostia of the right-sided pulmonary veins on the right side of the monitor (Figure 17C).

By both these maneuvers, it is possible to obtain an en face of ASD which is shown in Figure 18. Here all the rims are seen and an adequate selection for the ASD Device to be used for the closure of the defect can made.

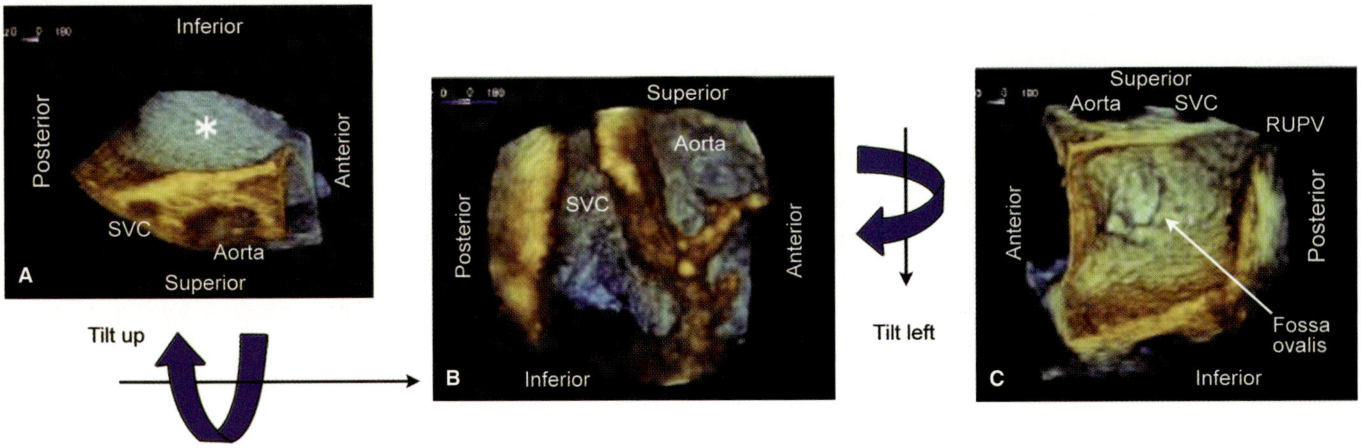

Figures 17 A, B, and C: (Adapted from Muhamed Saric, JASE 2010;23:1128-35)

A : Shows the 3D TEE picture of normal inter atrial septum viewed at 0 Degrees Horizontal Axis. The SVC is seen on the right atrial side and the Ascending Aorta is seen on the left atrial side. These structures are important landmarks and have to be properly identified and oriented in correct anatomical position

B: TUPLE I : The image in 17 A is Tilted up

C: TUPLE II : The image is leftward rotated

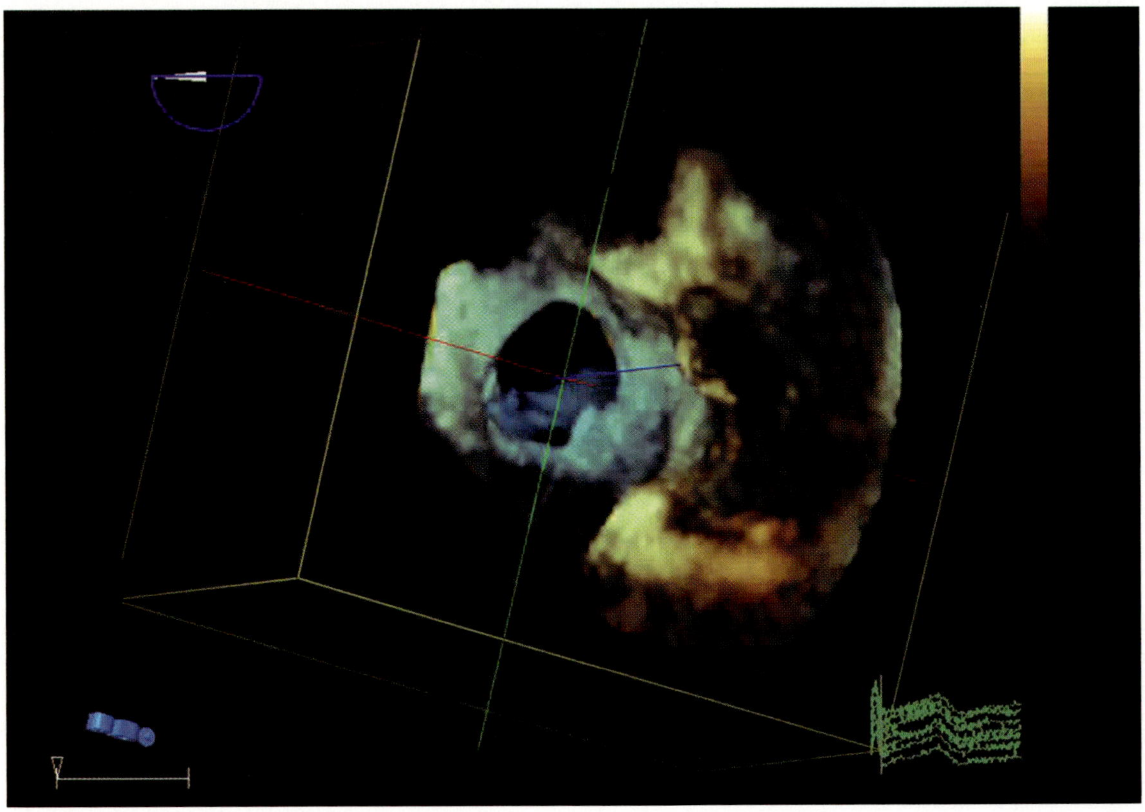

Figure 18: The 3D Full volume view of the ASD after the TUPLE manoveurs as viewed from the left atrial side. Note all the rims are visible

CLINICAL IMPLICATIONS OF RT3D-TEE

Real-time 3D-MTEE consistently provides excellent quality volume rendered images of mitral valve components, including anterior and posterior leaflets, as well as annulus and subvalvular structures, as evidenced by the high visualization scores. This finding suggests that 3D-MTEE imaging may become one of the modalities of choice to assess this valve during peri operative planning of MV surgery. The IAS and LAA are also well visualized because both structures are relatively posteriorly located.

Transesophageal 3D echocardiography thus far has had the major disadvantage that reconstruction was performed offline. It was thus used mostly for scientific investigations. An RT3D-TEE system with good spatial and temporal resolution, however, has great potential for numerous clinical applications. This applies both for already-established procedures and for new ones currently under development. For example, navigation of the catheter for electrophysiological studies has been performed thus far with fluoroscopy. On the one hand, the examiner only obtains a 2D summation image of the cardiac structures in this procedure. On the other hand, procedures like the ablation of atrial fibrillation are accompanied by extensive radiation. Transesophageal real-time 3D echocardiography could thus become an important supplement to imaging in electrophysiology. It would also be a valuable procedure for controlling the intervention in percutaneous implantations of ASD occluders or cardiac valves. The development of new surgical procedures in the future should enable operations like ASD occlusion or mitral valve repair on the beating heart under 3D echocardiographic control.

REFERENCES

1. Judy Hung, Roberto Lang, Frank Flachskampf, et al. 3D echocardiography: A review of the current status and future directions. ASE position paper. JASE Nov 2007.
2. Kuberan Pushparajah, Owen I Miller, John M Simpson. 3D echocardiography of the atrial septum anatomical features and landmarks for the echocardiographer. JACC: Cardiovascular imaging. 2010;3(9).
3. Arthur E Weyman. The year in echocardiography. JACC January 7, 2004;43(1):140-8.
4. Michael Handke, Gudrun Heinrichs, Urs Moser, et al. Transesophageal real-time three-dimensional echocardiography. Methods and initial in vitro and human in vivo studies. J Am Coll Cardiol 2006;48:2070-6.
5. Lissa Sugeng, Stanton K Shernan, Ivan S Salgo, et al. Live 3-dimensional transesophageal echocardiography initial experience using the fully-sampled matrix array probe. Am Coll Cardiol 2008;52:446-9.
6. Victor Mor-Avi, Lissa Sugeng, Roberto M Lang. Real-time 3-dimensional echocardiography. An integral component of the routine echocardiographic examination in adult patients? Circulation 2009;119:314-29.
7. Bhan A, Kapetanakis S and Monaghan MJ. Three-dimensional echocardiography. Heart 2010;96:153-63.
8. Amer M Johri, Jonathan J Passeri, Michael H Picard. Three-dimensional echocardiography: approaches and clinical utility. Heart 2010;96:390-7.
9. Francesco F Faletra, Siew Y Ho, P Angelo Auricchio. Anatomy of right atrial structures by real-time 3D transesophageal echocardiography. JACC: Cardio imaging. Sep 2010;3(3): 966-75.
10. Alan S Pearlman. Echocardiography 2020: Opportunities and Challenges. JASE. August 2010;23(8).
11. Decebal Gabriel Latcu, Jean-Paul Rinaldi, Nadir Saoudi. Real-time three-dimensional transoesophageal echocardiography for diagnosis of left atrial appendage thrombus. European Journal of Echocardiography 2009;10:711-2.
12. Cezary Szmigielski, Kashif Rajpoot, Vicente Grau, et al. Real-time 3D fusion echocardiography. J Am Coll Cardiol Img 2010;3:682-90.
13. Jan N Hilberath, Daryl A Oakes, Stanton K Shernan, et al. Safety of transesophageal echocardiography. J Am Soc Echocardiogr 2010;23:1115-27.
14. Franke A, Rulands D, Breithardt OA, et al. Transthoracic high-resolution real-time three-dimensional echocardiography for the analysis of regional left-ventricular wall motion patterns in patients with cardiac resynchronization therapy. European Heart Journal Vol 24, Abstr. Suppl. August/September 2003, p. 396.
15. Kapetenakis S, Murray O, Rance K, et al. Contrast enhanced real-time three-dimensional echocardiography, is it feasible? European Heart Journal, Abstr. Suppl. August/September 2003;24:700.
16. Kühl HP, Rulands D, Schreckenberg M, et al. Assessment of left-ventricular volumes and function using high-resolution transthoracic real-time three-dimensional echocardiography: comparison of semi-automatic border detection with manual contour tracing. European Heart Journal, Abstr. Suppl. August/September 2003;24:352.

17. Marx G. The real deal: Real-time 3D echocardiography in congenital heart disease. Pediatric Cardiology Today. September 2003;1(1):9-11.
18. Shirali G. Live 3D echo clarifies anatomy of recurrent subaortic stenosis and a shadow in the left atrium. RT Image. June 23, 2003;16(25).
19. Lang R, Sugeng L. A fantastic journey: 3D cardiac ultrasound goes live. Radiology Management. 2002 Nov-Dec;24(6):18-22.
20. Ahmad M, Xie T, Chamoun AJ, et al. Images in cardiovascular medicine. Real-time three-dimensional echocardiography with real-time volume rendering in assessment of left ventricular apical thrombi. Circulation. 2002 Sep 24;106(13):e53.
21. Belohlavek M, Tanabe K, Jakrapanichakul D, et al. Rapid three-dimensional echocardiography: clinically feasible alternative for precise and accurate measurement of left ventricular volumes. Circulation. 2001 Jun 19;103(24):2882-4.
22. Qin JX, Shiota T, McCarthy PM, Firstenberg MS, Greenberg NL, Tsujino H, Bauer F, Travaglini A, Hoercher KJ, Buda T, Smedira NG, Thomas JD. Investigator: Thomas JD. Real-time three-dimensional echocardiographic study of left ventricular function after infarct exclusion surgery for ischemic cardiomyopathy. Circulation. 2000 Nov 7;102(19 Suppl 3): III101-6.
23. Yao J, Cao QL, Masani N, et al. Three-dimensional echocardiographic estimation of infarct mass based on quantification of dysfunctional left ventricular mass. Circulation. 1997 Sep 2;96(5):1660-6.
24. Hung J, Guerrero JL, Handschumacher MD, et al. Reverse ventricular remodeling reduces ischemic mitral regurgitation: Echo-guided device application in the beating heart. Circulation. 12 Nov 2002;106(20):2594-2600.
25. Kwan J, Shiota T, Agler DA, et al. Real-time three-dimensional echocardiography study. Geometric differences of the mitral apparatus between ischemic and dilated cardiomyopathy with significant mitral regurgitation: real-time three-dimensional echocardiography study. Circulation. 2003 Mar 4;107(8):1135-40.
26. Salgo IS, Gorman JH 3rd, Gorman RC, et al. Effect of annular shape on leaflet curvature in reducing mitral leaflet stress. Circulation. 2002 Aug 6;106(6):711-7.
27. Buck T, Mucci RA, Guerrero JL, et al. The power-velocity integral at the vena contracta: A new method for direct quantification of regurgitant volume flow. Circulation. 2000 Aug 29;102(9):1053-61.
28. Qin JX, Shiota T, Lever HM, Rubin DN, Bauer F, Kim YJ, Sitges M, Greenberg NL, Drinko JK, Martin M, Agler DA, Thomas JD. Investigator: Thomas JD. Impact of left ventricular outflow tract area on systolic outflow velocity in hypertrophic cardiomyopathy: a real-time three-dimensional echocardiographic study. Journal of the American College of Cardiology. 2002 Jan 16;39(2):308-14.
29. Otsuji Y, Handschumacher MD, Liel-Cohen N, et al. Mechanism of ischemic mitral regurgitation with segmental left ventricular dysfunction: three-dimensional echo-cardiographic studies in models of acute and chronic progressive regurgitation. Journal of the American College of Cardiology. 2001 Feb;37(2):641-8.
30. Magni G, Hijazi ZM, Pandian NG, et al. Two- and three-dimensional transesophageal echocardiography in patient selection and assessment of atrial septal defect closure by the new DAS-Angel Wings device: initial clinical experience. Circulation. 1997 Sep 16;96(6):1722-8.
31. Marx GR, Sherwood MC. Three-dimensional echo-cardiography in congenital heart disease: a continuum of unfulfilled promises? No. A presently clinically applicable technology with an important future? Yes. [Review] [122 refs] Pediatric Cardiology. 2002 May-Jun;23(3):266-85.
32. Pedra CA, Yoo SJ, Soderberg B, et al. Aneurysm of the membranous septum in critical pulmonary stenosis: spontaneous rupture after balloon dilatation. Pediatric Cardiology. 2001 Jul-Aug;22(4):359-62.
33. Subahi SA. Distinguishing cardiac features of a novel form of congenital muscular dystrophy (Salih cmd). Pediatric Cardiology. 2001 Jul-Aug;22(4):297-301.
34. McElhinney DB, Hoydu AK, Gaynor JW, et al. Patterns of right aortic arch and mirror-image branching of the brachiocephalic vessels without associated anomalies. Pediatric Cardiology. 2001 Jul-Aug;22(4):285-91.
35. Muhamed Saric, Gila Perk MD, Jan R, et al. Imaging atrial septal defects by real-time three-dimensional transesophageal echocardiography: Step-by-Step Approach JASE 2010;23:1128-35.

CHAPTER 3

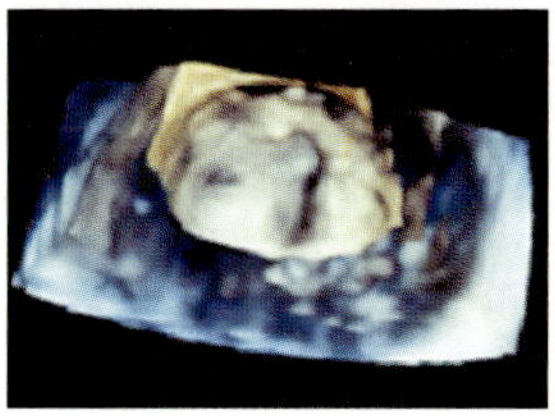

Three-Dimensional Echocardiographic Evaluation of Patients with Rheumatic Mitral Stenosis

V Amuthan, GS Siva Kumar

3D TOPOGRAPHY OF THE MITRAL VALVE

The mitral valve is a complex structure three dimentionally consisting of atrioventricular junction or the mitral annulus, anterior and posterior mitral leaflets with commissures in medial and lateral aspects, Chordae Tendinae, anterolateral and posteromedial papillary muscles and the ventricular myocardial attachments (Figure 1).[1] 3D echocardiography both transthoracic and transesophageal have the power to view the mitral valve from the left atrium. Table 1 illustrates the tips and tricks of acquiring a good live 3D image. This surgeon's view (described in chapter 2), shows that the anterior and posterior mitral leaflets have several indentations dividing them into segments or scallops. The anterior leaflet has three scallops: A1 – anterolateral, A2 – middle, A3 – posteromedial. Similarly, the posterior leaflet has three scallops: P1 – anterolateral, P2 – middle, P3 – posteromedial, Figures 2 to 5 show the anterior mitral leaflet and the posterior mitral leaflet scallops as they are seen in long axis, short axis, apical 4 chamber and apical 2 chamber views. The anterior and posterior leaflets are fused for 3 to 8 mm medially and laterally at the trigones and usually form distinct commissures (anterolateral and posteromedial). The anterior leaflet comprises roughly two thirds of the valve area, is about two-fold longer than the posterior leaflet, and is somewhat triangular. The posterior leaflet is more elongated and rectangular. The anterior leaflet is attached to the septum and fibrous annulus of the heart, and it is relatively nondistensible. Although the anterior leaflet accounts for two-thirds of the mitral valve area, its attachment to the mitral annulus accounts for only approximately one-third of the mitral annular circumference. The anterior mitral leaflet spans the distance between the two fibrous trigones and is in direct continuity with the noncoronary aortic valve leaflet. The posterior mitral valve leaflet is attached to the posterior two-thirds of the mitral annulus, which runs along the free wall of the left ventricle and is primarily muscular with little fibrous tissue explaining its tendency to distend and elongate.[1,2]

MITRAL STENOSIS

The severity of mitral stenosis is assessed mainly by estimation of the mitral valve area. Currently, the available 2D echocardiographic and Doppler techniques have their well-known limitations. The advent of 3D echocardiography has refined the assessment of mitral valve area to such an extent that today it is considered as a gold standard. Besides, 3D echocardiography has introduced new indices which further improve the diagnosis of mitral stenosis. By means of 3D echocardiography it is possible to assess the morphology of the mitral valve. It is also useful during balloon mitral valvuloplasty to assess the mechanism and success of the procedure.

ASSESSMENT OF MITRAL VALVE AREA

In a 3D homogeneous data set using any plane 3D echocardiography, it is possible to pinpoint the cut plane to the tips of the mitral valve so the true anatomic valve area can be measured (Figure 6). Table 1 illustrates the use of Q Lab protocol for measuring the mitral valve area accurately. The advantage of this method is, contrary to 2D echocardiography, that proper alignment of the cut plane is controlled in a 3D data set. It is important because errors due to malpositioning can be obviated. It has been shown that malpositioning errors can achieve up to 88% (1.5 cm^2) in the measurement of the mitral valve area that is not acceptable in the management of patient with mitral stenosis.

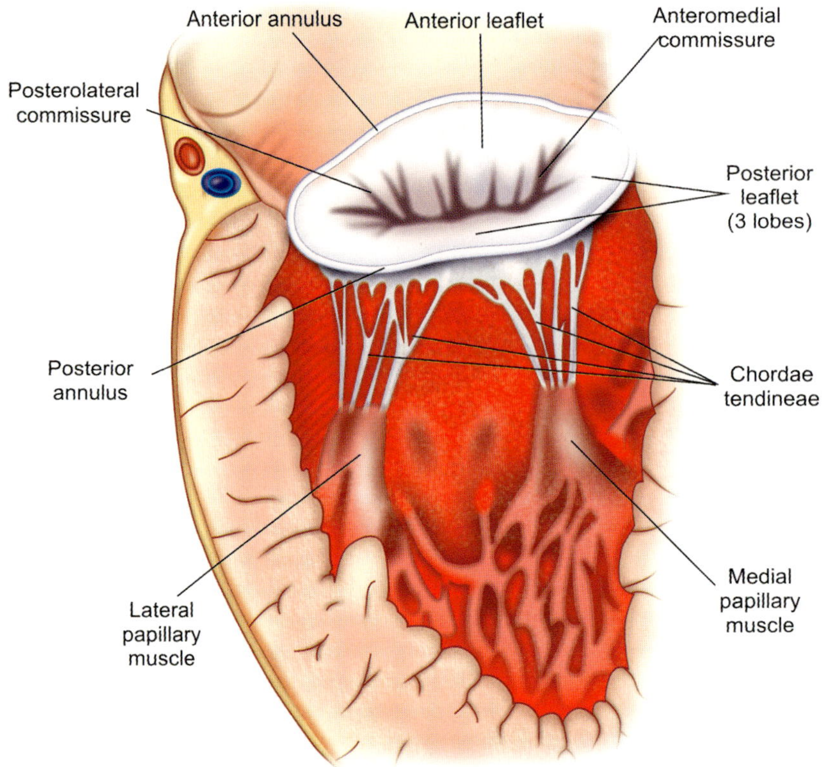

Figure 1: The Mitral valve apparatus. The mitral valve apparatus consists of the following: 1. The mitral annulus; 2. The mitral valves consisting of the anterior mitral leaflet (Scallops A1, A2, and A3 from lateral to medial) and posterior mitral leaflet (Scallops P1, P2 and P3) from lateral to medial. The leaflets are fused in the lateral aspect, which is called as lateral commisure and medially, which is called as the medial commissure; 3. The subvalvular apparatus consisting of the *Chordae tendineae*; 4. The papillary muscles: Anterolateral and posteromedial papillary muscles; 5. The ventricular attachment of the papillary muscles

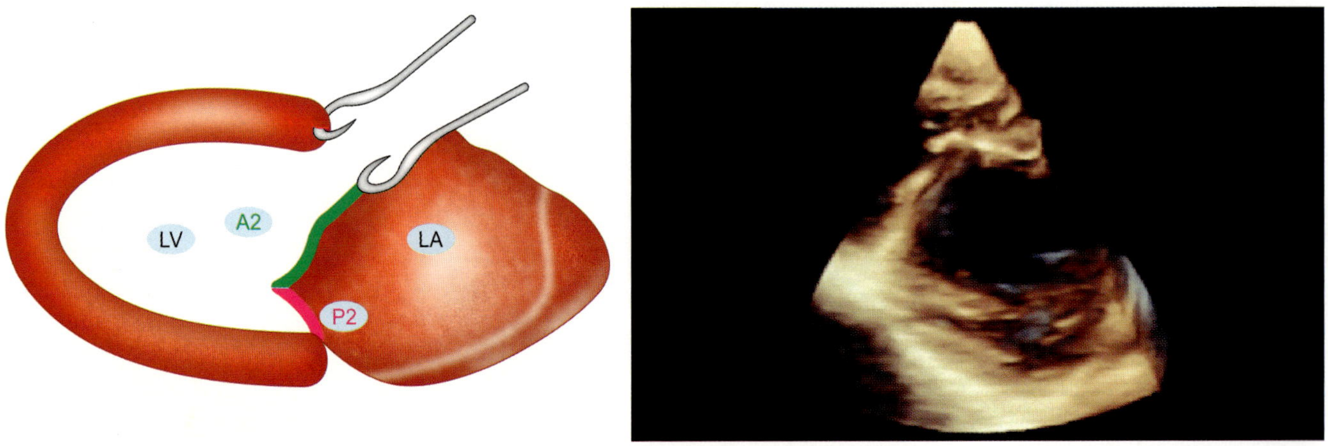

Figure 2: Parasternal long axis in rheumatic mitral stenosis: The left panel shows the diagram depicting the A2 and P2 of anterior mitral leaflet and posterior mitral leaflet. The leaflets are thickened in mitral stenosis with commissural fusion and calcification. The pathology also extends to the subvalvular apparatus with thickening and fusion of *Chordae tendineae*. All these lead to the reduction in valve area in the rheumatic mitral stenosis (Diagram adapted from European Society of Cardiology)

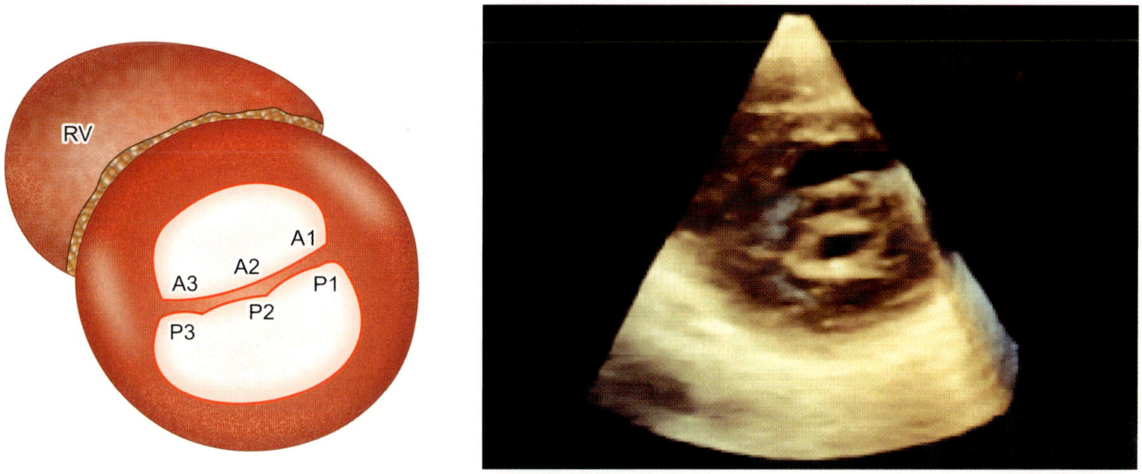

Figure 3: Parasternal short axis in rheumatic mitral stenosis: This plane is ideally suited for the calculation of valve area in 2D echocardiography. Live 3D examination adds another dimension to this. This helps to identify A1, A2 and A3 of AML and P1, P2, and P3 of PML from lateral to medial aspect. This view is ideally suited to have a look at the medial and lateral commissures, especially after balloon mitral commissurotomy (Diagram adapted from European Society of Cardiology)

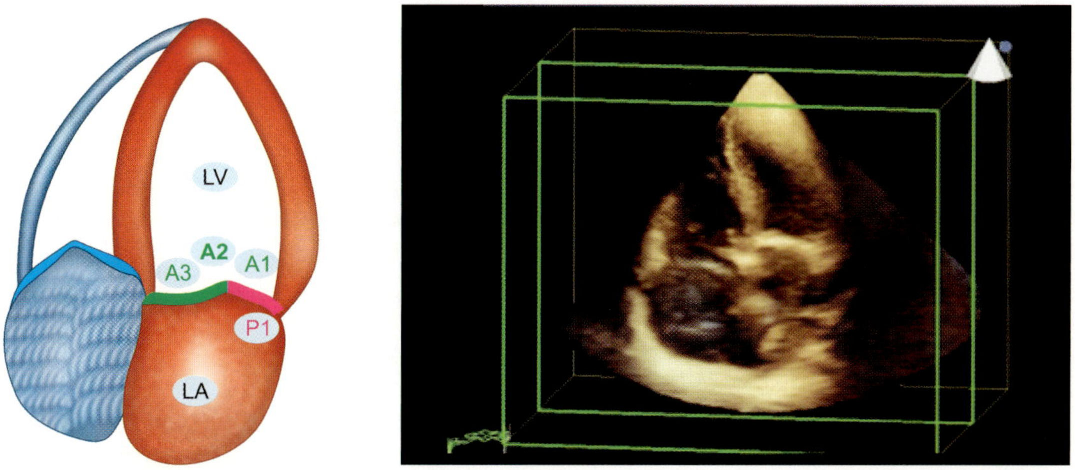

Figure 4: Apical 4 chamber view: This view is ideally suited for acquiring the Live 3D slice (Narrow slice 3D) and full volume trace. After acquiring the image 3D Q mitral valve analysis is done (Diagram adapted from European Society of Cardiology)

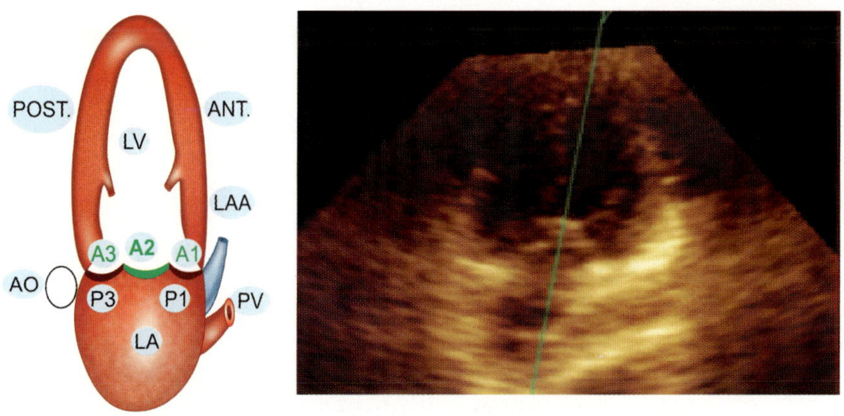

Figure 5: Apical 2 chamber plane showing the mitral valve leaflet P3, A3, A2, A1 and P1 (Diagram adapted from European Society of Cardiology)

In addition, assessment of the anatomic mitral valve area is advantageous because it is hemodynamically independent. This is in contrast to effective mitral valve area (measured by pressure half-time and PISA methods) which is hemodynamically influenced by associated abnormalities (aortic insufficiency and increased left ventricular stiffness). In the first studies carried out by Kupferwasser et al and Chen et al, the mitral valve area was assessed by any plane 3D transesophageal echocardiography (TEE).[3-5] Figure 7 illustrates the Trans Esophageal echocardiographic appearances of mitral stenosis in the horizontal plane (Panel A), from left atrial side (Panel B), short axis view (panel C), bicommissural view (Panel D) and long axis view (Panel E). The mitral valve area assessed by 3D echocardiography was compared with the mitral valve area measured by 2D methods (2D planimetry and pressure half-time) and invasively assessed mitral valve area according to the Gorlin formula. Only Kasliwal et al compared the mitral valve areas by 3D echocardiography with the true mitral orifice measured directly at operation.

The comparison achieved a high degree of agreement with 3D echocardiography.[6] Thus, 3D echocardiography, today, can be considered as a new clinical standard in the assessment of the anatomic mitral valve area. 3D echocardiography also

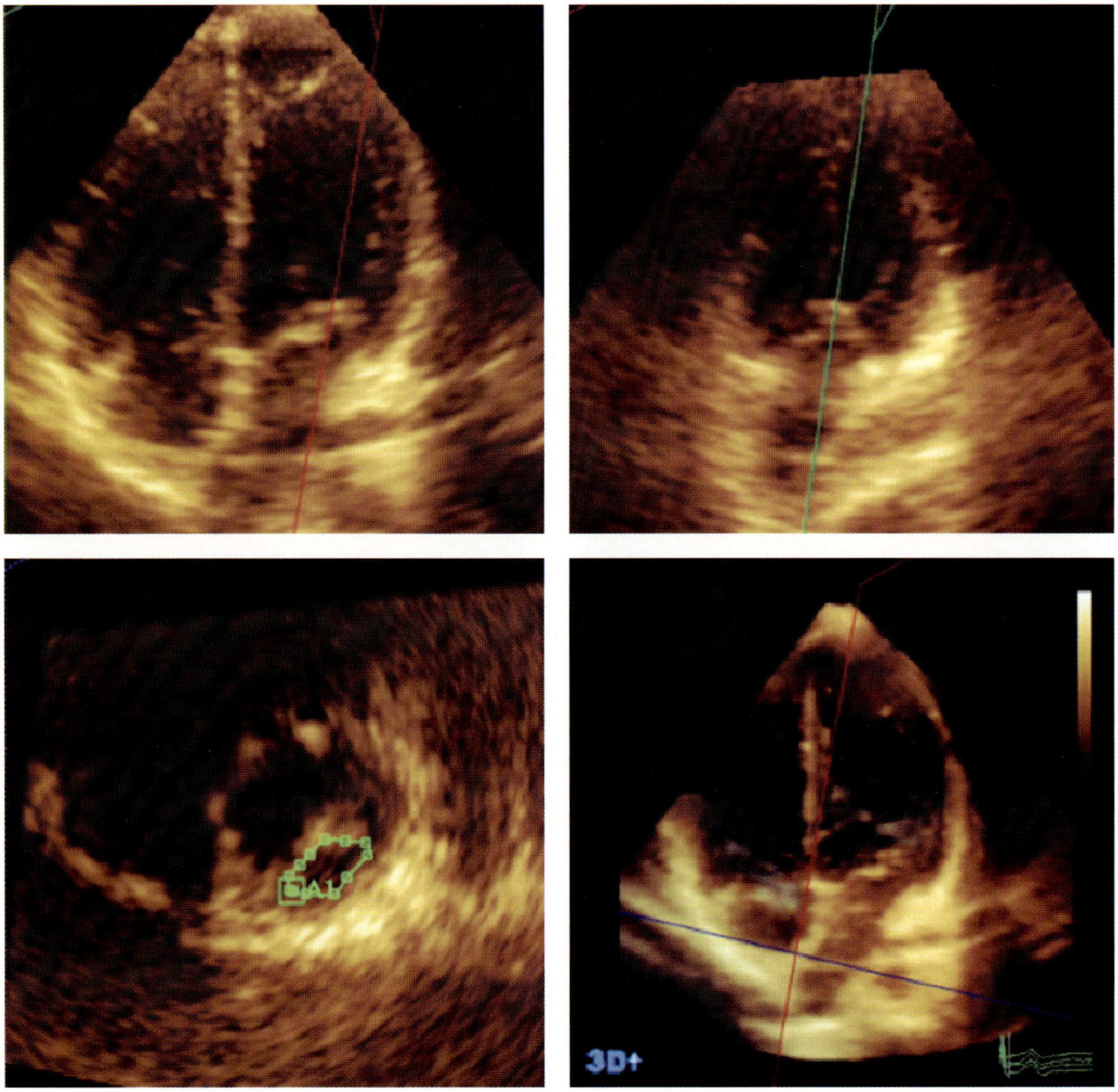

Figure 6: 3D Quantification of mitral valve

TABLE 1 Live 3D: Imaging the mitral valve and mitral valve Q Lab protocol

Live 3D Zoom (Benefit: immediate result and ECG triggering not necessary)

- Use four chamber, two chamber, or long axis views
- Optimize image and reduce near field TGC in 2D (to reduce LA haze)
- Adjust zoom box size and position to include entire annulus in the zoom box (and aortic root if wanting to use MVQ plug-in) Remember increasing box size reduces frame rate
- Line density control balances image quality and frame rate: low line density = higher frame rate but reduced IQ and vice versa
- Check 2D Opts and gain in 3D to find best 3D image and acquire

3D Full Volume (Benefit: higher frame rate and better IQ)

- Use four chamber or two chamber views
- Optimize 2D image, reduce depth, and reduce near field gain
- Adjust density and Fv Opt as necessary
- Acquire using breathhold

MVQ Protocol

Note: This is listed at top left of screen. Hovering over each step will provide a brief explanation and highlight necessary controls. Clicking on the protocol step or the tools list will activate tools. As points are edited and measurements completed they turn from red to green

- Find and tag ES (end systolic) frame
- Align MPRs and model:
  - In red quad rotate image so aortic valve and root can be seen clearly on left to image
  - Line up blue plane in red and green quad so it sits just above mitral annular level and parallel to it. Align green plane in red quad and red plane in green quad so that they intersect the mitral valve at the midpoint
  - Check in blue quad that red and green planes cut across the short axis of the annulus maximum diameter
  - Rotate model in bottom right quad to match 3D volume orientation (Pull volume towards you to be able to see MV)
- Select protocol level: Click on preferences to select protocol level you wish to perform (basic, standard or advanced). Number of slices will change automatically. This can be a manually changed as well. Also ensure sticky clicks and navigation tools are checked on and required measurements selected
- Add reference points: Place annular points at insertion of leaflet into annulus following a left to right workflow
- Edit nadir and aortic point: Place Ao point at insertion of non-coronary cusp into aortic annulus. Edit nadir point (lowest point of mitral valve into the LV)
- Edit annulus points: Use navigate tools to move between slices for standard or advanced model
- Edit commissural points on the blue plane watching the red plane changing as a reference to identify and position the commissural points
- Trace leaflet: Clicking on this step will enlarge red quad. Left click to start tracing and left click to end. Use the navigate tools to advance through slices. If a cooptation point appears on the slice click on the icon at top right of quad to show the break between the leaflets, and position the height to demonstrate the regurgitant orifice. Click on R quad next to MPR mode button on panel to return to viewing all four quads
- Edit cooptation and border points: In the blue plane click on the diamonds and reposition to define the leaflet segments
- Find and add papillary tips (if seen): use the navigate keys in the blue plane to move the plane down until the papillary tips can be seen and label anterolateral and Posteromedial tips

has been shown to be accurate in the assessment of mitral valve area by transthoracic approach. Sugeng et al[6,7] confirmed that free-hand 3D transthoracic echocardiography comparing with 2D planimetry, pressure half-time and the PISA methods is the most accurate when it was compared with invasively determined mitral valve area according to the Gorlin formula. The most attractive is definitely RT3D echocardiography which allows on-line assessment of the mitral valve area. Images are displayed as two simultaneous intersecting orthogonal long-axis scans (B-mode scans) and two perpendicular short-axis scans (C-mode scans). These C-mode scans allow the display of short-axis views of the mitral valve from an apical transducer position. Binder et al found out that RT3D echocardiography comparing with 2D planimetry and pressure half-time methods allows accurate measurement of the mitral valve area from the transthoracic

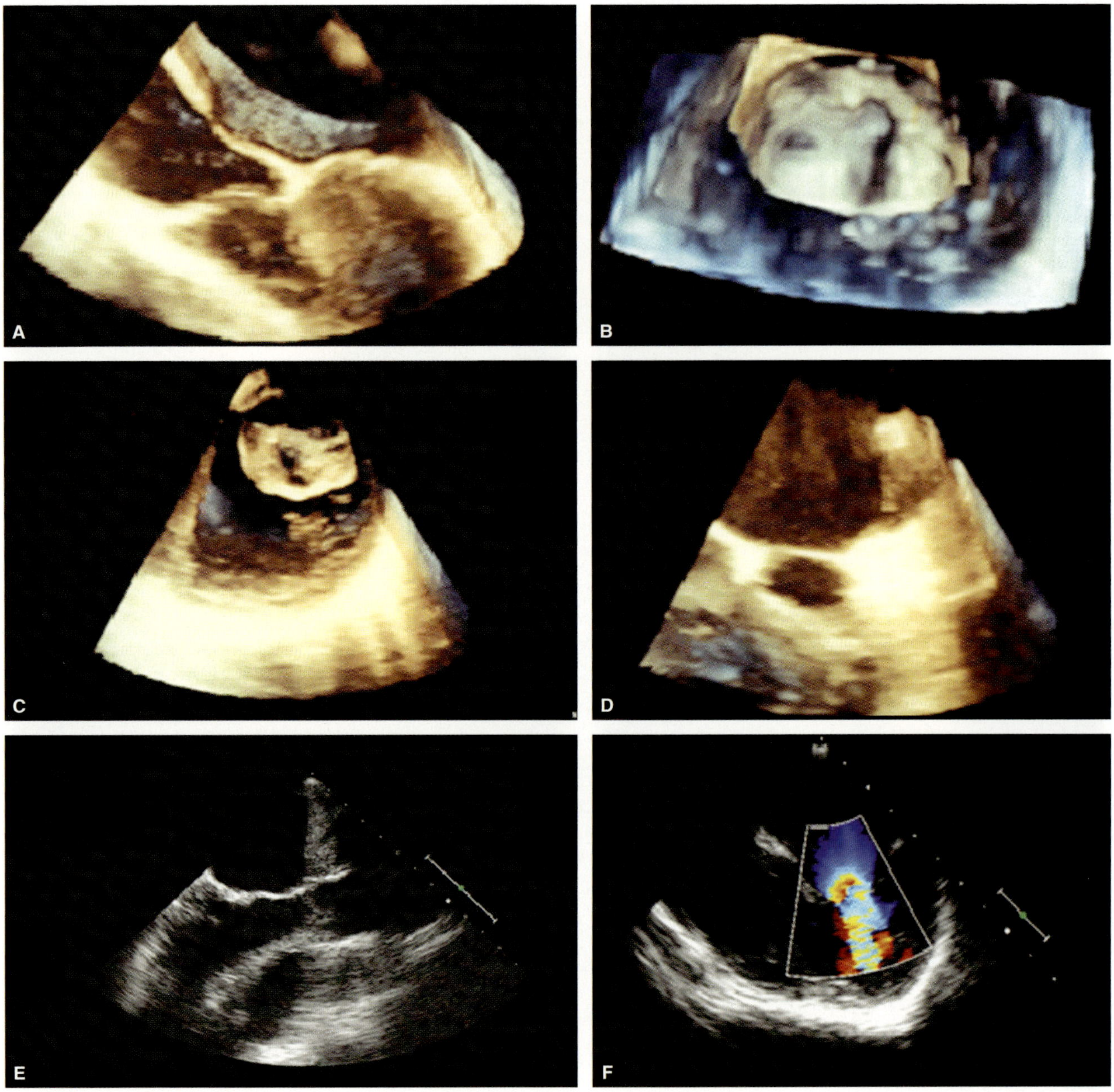

Figure 7: 3D TEE image of mitral stenosis: Panel A horizontal view in the four chamber plane. Panel B shows 3D Echo from the left atrial side. Panel C shows short axis view from the left atrial side. Panel D shows bicommissural view. Panel E shows TEE long axis view at 120 degrees. Panel F shows TEE horizontal plane color flow MS Jet

approach.[6,7] It is evident in patients with an adequate acoustic window.

NEW INDICES OF MITRAL STENOSIS

Thickening of mitral leaflets in rheumatic mitral stenosis is a well-known phenomenon. Limbu et al were the first who quantified the mitral valve volume *in vivo* in normal subjects and patients with rheumatic mitral stenosis. The mitral valve volume in normal individuals was on average 4.5 ml and in patients with mitral stenosis 9 ml. When they divided patients with mitral stenosis into the sinus rhythm and atrial fibrillation groups, patients with atrial fibrillation had a propensity to have a larger mitral valve volume and were older than patients with sinus rhythm. Thus, etiologic

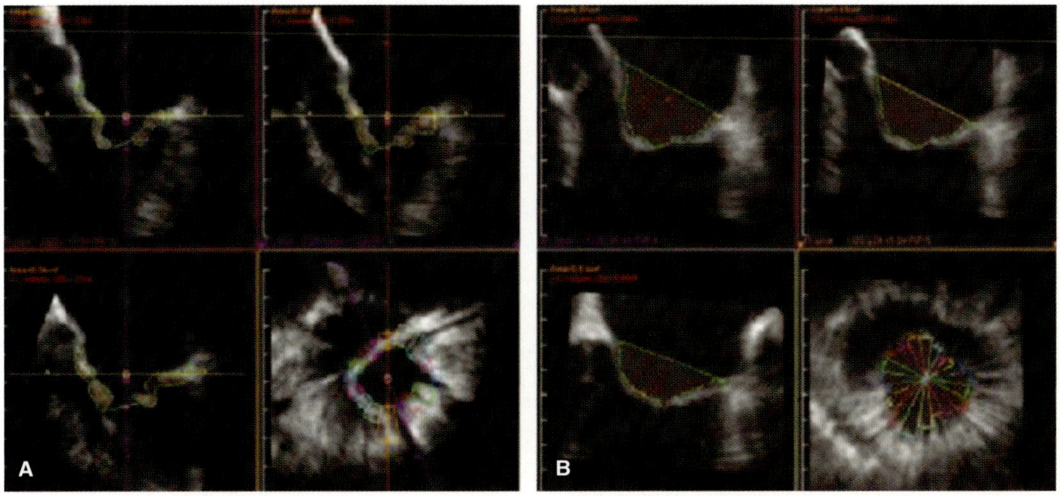

Figures 8A and B: (A) Mitral valve volume measurement, (B) Mitral valve doming volume measurement

TABLE 2 Echocardiographic score to assess outcome of balloon valvuloplasty

Grade	*Mobility*	*Subvalvular thickening*	*Thickening*	*Calcification*
1.	Highly mobile valve with only leaflet tips restricted	Minimal thickening just below the mitral leaflets	Leaflets near normal in thickness (4 to 5 mm)	A single area of increased echo brightness
2.	Leaflet mid and base portions have normal mobility	Thickening of chordal structures extending up to one-third of chordal length	Midleaflets normal, considerable thickening of margins (5 to 8 mm)	Scattered areas of brightness confined to leaflet margins
3.	Valve continues to move forward in diastole, mainly from the base	Thickening extending to the distal third of the chords	Thickening extending through the entire leaflet (5 to 8 mm)	Brightness extending into the midportion of the leaflets
4.	No or minimal forward movement of the leaflets in diastole	Extensive thickening and shortening of all chordal structures extending down to the papillary muscles	Considerable thickening of all leaflet tissue (greater than 8 to 10 mm)	Extensive brightness throughout much of the leaflet tissue

relationship between atrial fibrillation and further enlargement of the mitral valve volume was speculated. Gilon et al studied *in vitro* the hypothesis that the stenotic mitral valve influences the pressures and flows not only by cross-sectional area but also by 3D geometry of the stenotic valve proximal to the orifice.[8] With the use of 3D echocardiography and stereolithography they constructed by laser polymerization different shapes of mitral valve: domed, intermediate and flattened. Coefficient of contraction was calculated as effective area divided by anatomic orifice area. Coefficient of contraction decreased as the mitral valve was flattened. The study confirmed, that variations in contraction coefficient (i.e. the 3D geometry of the mitral valve) led to varying pressure gradients that were up to 40% higher for the flattest valves. Thus, doming valves permit a higher cardiac output than flat ones.

3D ECHOCARDIOGRAPHY IN BALLOON MITRAL VALVULOPLASTY (TABLE 2)

3D echocardiography by volume rendering allows visualization of the mitral valve en face either from the left atrium or the left ventricle.[8,9] Applebaum et al evaluated the mechanism of balloon valvuloplasty by 3D echocardiography.[16] Volume rendered 3D images enabled visualization of commissural splitting and leaflet tears not seen on 2D. They found that balloon mitral valvuloplasty was more successful when complete splitting was achieved as compared with partial splitting. Moreover, in 38% of patients in whom an increase of mitral regurgitation developed, tear was visualized by 3D. One group, Langerveld et al conducted a similar study where 3D TEE enabled a better description of the mitral valvular anatomy following balloon mitral valvuloplasty, comparing to 2D echocardiography. In addition, significant relation of mitral valve volume before valvuloplasty to a successful procedure was found. A new index, the doming volume, which allows quantification of the mobility and three dimensional goemetry of the mitral valve has also been described (Figures 8A and B). Patients with a flat geometry of the mitral valve have a propensity to atrial fibrillation. Mitral valve volume can be used for quantitative evaluation of mitral stenosis and tends to be greater in patients with critical stenosis. Three-dimensional TEE can provide additional information to 2D TTE in patients with mitral stenosis, pre-percutaneous mitral valvuloplasty and post-percutaneous mitral valvuloplasty.[9,10] It can be a valuable alternative when mitral valve area assessment by 2D trans thoracic echocardiography is not reliable. The mitral valve volume can be assessed by 3D TEE. The MVV is inversely correlated to a successful PTMV procedure and can possibly be useful for the selection of patients for PTMV. Post-PTMV 3D TEE improves the description of the valvular anatomy. This enables more understanding of the mechanisms of successful PTMV and its complications. Both technical improvement and larger studies are needed before the usefulness of 3D TEE in patients with MVS is clear.

CONCLUSION

In summary, although the 3D-TEE probe allows excellent visualization of native MVs, LAA, IAS, and pulmonic veins, consistent optimal imaging of the AV and TVs may require further technological advances. Optimal visualization of MV apparatus components may allow quantification of its complex geometry and thus improve the diagnostic accuracy of echocardiographic evaluation of the MV. Overall, the ease and speed of data acquisition coupled with the ability to display cardiac structures using unique 3D views is likely to result in rapid integration of 3D Trans Esophageal Echocardiography into clinical practice. The accompanying video - (Chapter 3 video 1) illustrates the advantages of 3D Echo and 3D TEE over 2D Echocardiography in the diagnosis of Mitral Stenosis Chapter 3 Video 2 illustrates the Q Lab quantification of Mitral stenosis.

REFERENCES

1. Salustri A, Becker AE, van HL, et al. Three-dimensional echocardiography of normal and pathologic mitral valve: a comparison with two- dimensional transesophageal echocardiography. J Am Coll Cardiol 1996;27:1502-10.
2. Seward JB, Khandheria BK, Oh JK, et al. Transesophageal echocardiography: technique, anatomic correlations, implementation, and clinical applications. Mayo Clin Proc 1988;63:649-80.
3. Pandian NG, Hsu TL, Schwartz SL, et al. Multiplane transesophageal echocardiography. Imaging planes, echocardiographic anatomy, and clinical experience with a prototype phased array OmniPlane probe. Echocardiography 1992;9:649-66.
4. Roelandt JR, Fraser AG. Transesophageal echocardiography: clinical applications and prospects. Curr Opin Cardiol 1990;5:783-94.
5. Roelandt JR, Thomson IR, Vletter WB, et al. Multiplane transesophageal echocardiography: latest evolution in an imaging revolution. J Am Soc Echocardiogr 1992;5: 361-7.
6. Salustri A, Roelandt J. Three dimensional reconstruction of the heart with rotational acquisition: methods and clinical applications. Br Heart J 1995;73:10-5.
7. Wang XF, Deng YB, Nanda NC, et al. Live three-dimensional echocardiography: imaging principles and clinical application. Echocardiography 2003;20:593-604.
8. Kuhl HP, Schreckenberg M, Rulands D, et al. High-resolution transthoracic real-time three-dimensional echocardiography: quantitation of cardiac volumes and function using semi-automatic border detection and comparison with cardiac magnetic resonance imaging. J Am Coll Cardiol 2004;43:2083-90.
9. Roelandt JR, ten Cate FJ, Vletter WB, et al. Ultrasonic dynamic three-dimensional visualization of the heart with a multiplane transesophageal imaging transducer. J Am Soc Echocardiogr 1994;7:217-29.
10. Ludomirsky A, Vermilion R, Nesser J, et al. Transthoracic real-time three-dimensional echocardiography using the rotational scanning approach for data acquisition. Echocardiography 1994;11:599-606.

CHAPTER 4

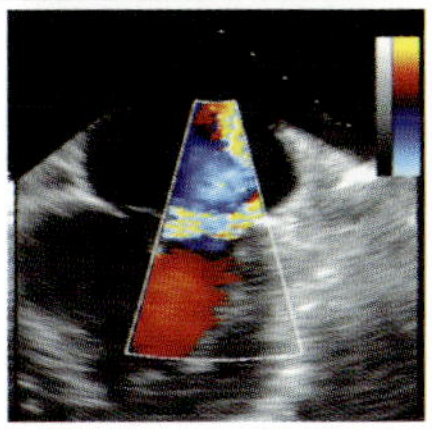

Three-Dimensional Echocardiography in Mitral Valve Regurgitation

V Amuthan, R Aravazhi, A Jegadeeswari, SR Veeramani

INTRODUCTION

Echocardiography remains the fastest, least expensive, and least invasive screening modality. The diagnostic capability of echocardiography has evolved dramatically over the last five decades from M-mode (1950s) to two-dimensional (2D) echocardiography (1970s). Though conventional 2D echocardiography is crucial to our understanding of the complex anatomy and spatial relationships of cardiac structures, it requires the mental integration of a limited number of 2D imaging planes which is inherently variable according to observer expertise.

Three-dimensional echocardiography (3DE) has been developed during the last 15 to 20 years. Within the last 10 years its clinical value has been proven in many publications around the world.[1,2] One important application of 3DE is its use for assessing valvular structures.[3-5] Especially in valvular heart disease it is important to understand the complex spatial geometry of the valves[6] and the subvalvular apparatus with its chordae and papillary muscles. Without 3DE, this assessment needs to be done as a kind of mental 3D reconstruction based on 2D echocardiography. 3DE does not require such a mental 3D reconstruction process and is not based on any geometrical assumptions. In addition, it greatly helps to communicate the echocardiographic findings to the cardiac surgeon.

Recent advances in three-dimensional (3D) echocardiography include the availability of real-time imaging. Three-dimensional imaging can be performed with both transesophageal and transthoracic probes and has been used in the operating room and during percutaneous balloon mitral commissurotomy. It has led to improved insight into the complex geometry of the mitral valve, the mechanisms of functional and ischemic MR, and the abnormalities in mitral valve prolapse, and infective endocarditis (Table 1).

Carpenter has classified the mitral valvular lesions according to the disease, valvular lesions and the type of valvular dysfunction, which are called as Carpentier's triad (Table 2). The type of valvular dysfunction is further summarized in Table 3. Three-dimensional echocardiogram is ideally suited for analysis of this kind.

Three-dimensional echo can also help guide surgical repair. Three-dimensional color-flow imaging of the proximal flow convergence region has been shown to be accurate in quantifying MR and has the theoretical advantages of not relying on the assumption of a hemispheric proximal convergence shape.

The acquisition of 3DE data sets for valvular assessment is done in two different ways: (1) with 3D TEE multiplane probes using the gating or reconstruction technique or (2) with matrix array transthoracic transducers (TTE) in real time[7] (RT3DE). Both 3DE acquisition methods are commercially available for several ultrasound systems from various vendors. Recent transducer developments have been done to miniaturize the matrix array real-time transducer into a transesophageal echo (TEE) endoscope.

MITRAL REGURGITATION 3D TEE RECONSTRUCTION METHOD

3DE greatly improved the assessment and understanding of valvular anatomy and function.[8-12] It can provide a detailed en face visualization of valve structures like leaflet scallops, prolapses, or commissures, for example, for a better preoperative assessment. With severe MR due to mitral valve prolapse, the location and extent of the prolapse by

TABLE 1 Showing the disease condition and the valvular structures which are involved

Etiology	*Affected valve level(s)*
Chronic coronary artery disease	LV, papillary muscles, annulus
Ischemic MR	Leaflets, chordae, annulus
Myxomatous degeneration	LV, papillary muscles, annulus
Mitral valve prolapse	Leaflets, chordae
Barlow's valve	Leaflets, chordae
Nonischemic dilated cardiomyopathy	AML, papillary muscles, LV
Rheumatic heart disease	Annulus, leaflets
Healed infective endocarditis	Anterior leaflet
Hypertrophic obstructive cardiomyopathy	Leaflets, annulus
Mitral annular calcification	Leaflets, chordae
Congenital	Leaflets, chordae
Connective tissue diseases	
Rheumatoid arthritis	
Systemic lupus erythematosus	
Antiphospholipid antibody syndrome	
Radiation	
Drug	
Ergotamines	
Methysergide	
Pergolide (fenfluramine, dexfenfluramine)	

TABLE 2 Carpentier 's pathophysiologic triad

- Disease (the underlying etiology)
- The lesions (e.g. chordal elongation or rupture, leaflet distention, annular, leaflet and/or papillary muscle calcification, and annular dilation)
- The dysfunction (defined according to the systolic position of the leaflet margins in relation to the annular plane)

TABLE 3 Carpentier's classification of valvular dysfunction

- **Type I:** Dysfunction implies normal leaflet motion with isolated annular dilation, leading to poor leaflet coaptation
- **Type II:** Dysfunction is defined by excess motion of the margin of a leaflet segment above the annular plane and is the most common type of dysfunction in degenerative MV disease
- **Type III:** Restricted motion of the leaflet margin, which can be further subdivided
- **Type IIIa:** Restriction of motion in both systole and diastole (usually due to fibrosis of the subvalvular apparatus)
- **Type IIIb:** Only in systole (which usually results from ventricular remodeling with papillary displacement and leaflet tethering)

3D echo have been compared to the surgical status. There has been an excellent correlation between the 3D echocardiographic localization of the prolapse and surgical inspection, and between the volume of prolapsing and surgically resected tissue. Thus, the 3D reconstruction echo method allows a precise localization and an accurate quantification of the prolapsing portion of the leaflets, thus providing refinements in the surgical planning of mitral valve repair and in the selection of candidates for this intervention.

TRANSTHORACIC REAL-TIME 3D ECHOCARDIOGRAPHY

RT3DE can provide a real-time 3D reconstruction or display of the beating heart and its valvular structures during the acquisition. For RT3DE, a parasternal or apical window shall be used. The anterior leaflet can be visualized best from a parasternal long-axis position. As the posterior leaflet has a much smaller excursion compared with the anterior leaflet,

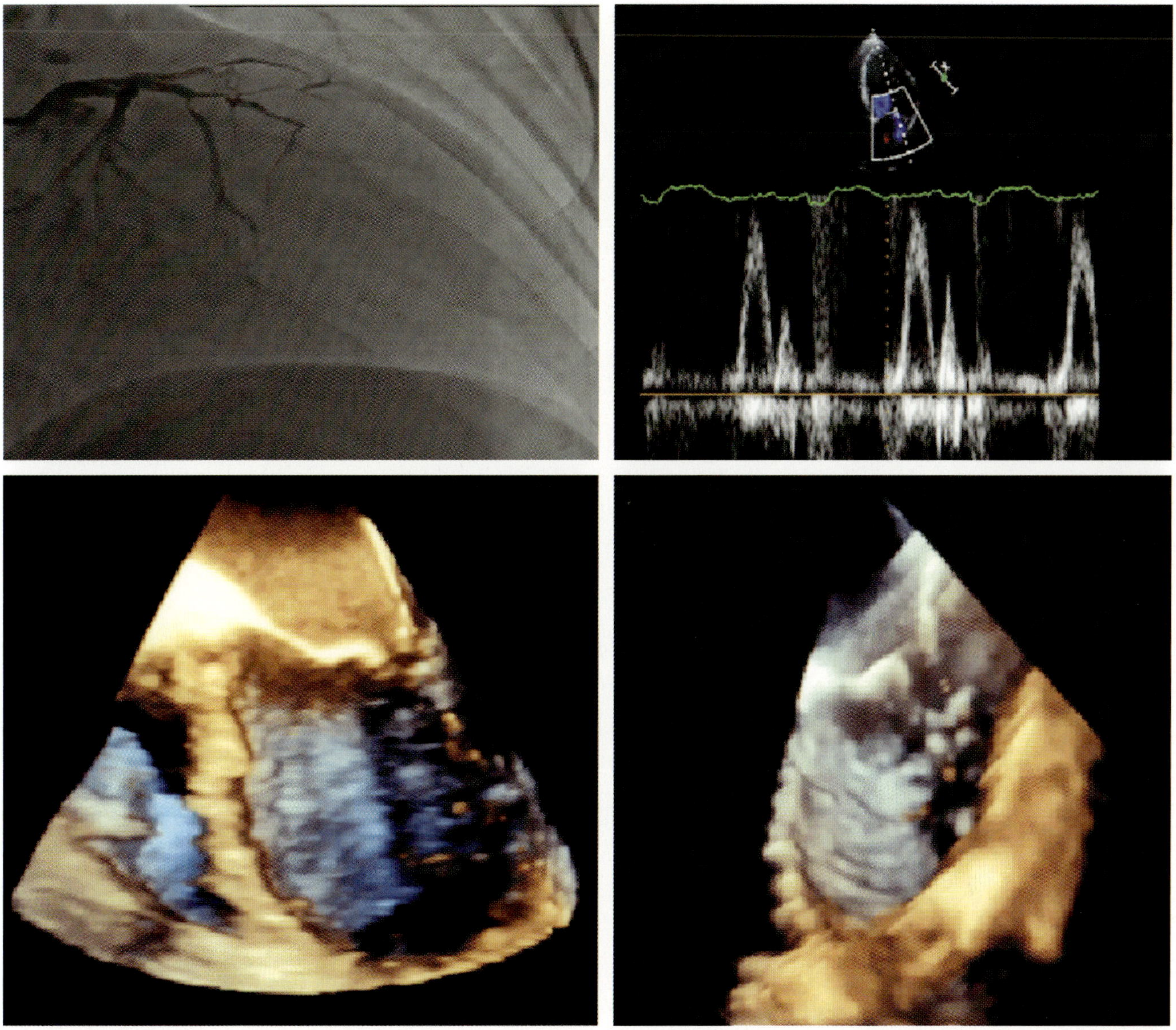

Figure 1: Ischemic MR in a patient with LBBB: Ischemic mitral regurgitation in a patient with acute coronary syndrome with LBBB . The top left panel showing coronary Angiogram with Osteoproximal disease of left anterior descending Artery and 99% Mid LAD and lesion in left circumflex. The Doppler echocardiography depicts mitral regurgitation and the 3D TEE showing incomplete systolic coaption in a dilated globally hypokinetic LV and normal mitral valve apparatus with dilated mitral annulus

it is sometimes more challenging to visualize. Then, an apical four-chamber position is preferable.

COLOR DOPPLER 3D ECHOCARDIOGRAPHY

Color Doppler 3D shows images of MR jet and flow convergence in patients with MR. TEE 3D reconstruction method discloses a larger paravalvular MR jet and the adherence of MR jet to the wall. The 3D en face images also demonstrate the exact location of the paravalvular leakage. Color Doppler 3D echocardiography can reveal unique views and can capture and demonstrate the entire jet to evaluate its direction and volume, which cannot be appreciated by multiple 2D echo views. Color 3D echocardiography can also demonstrate dynamic changes in the MR jet.

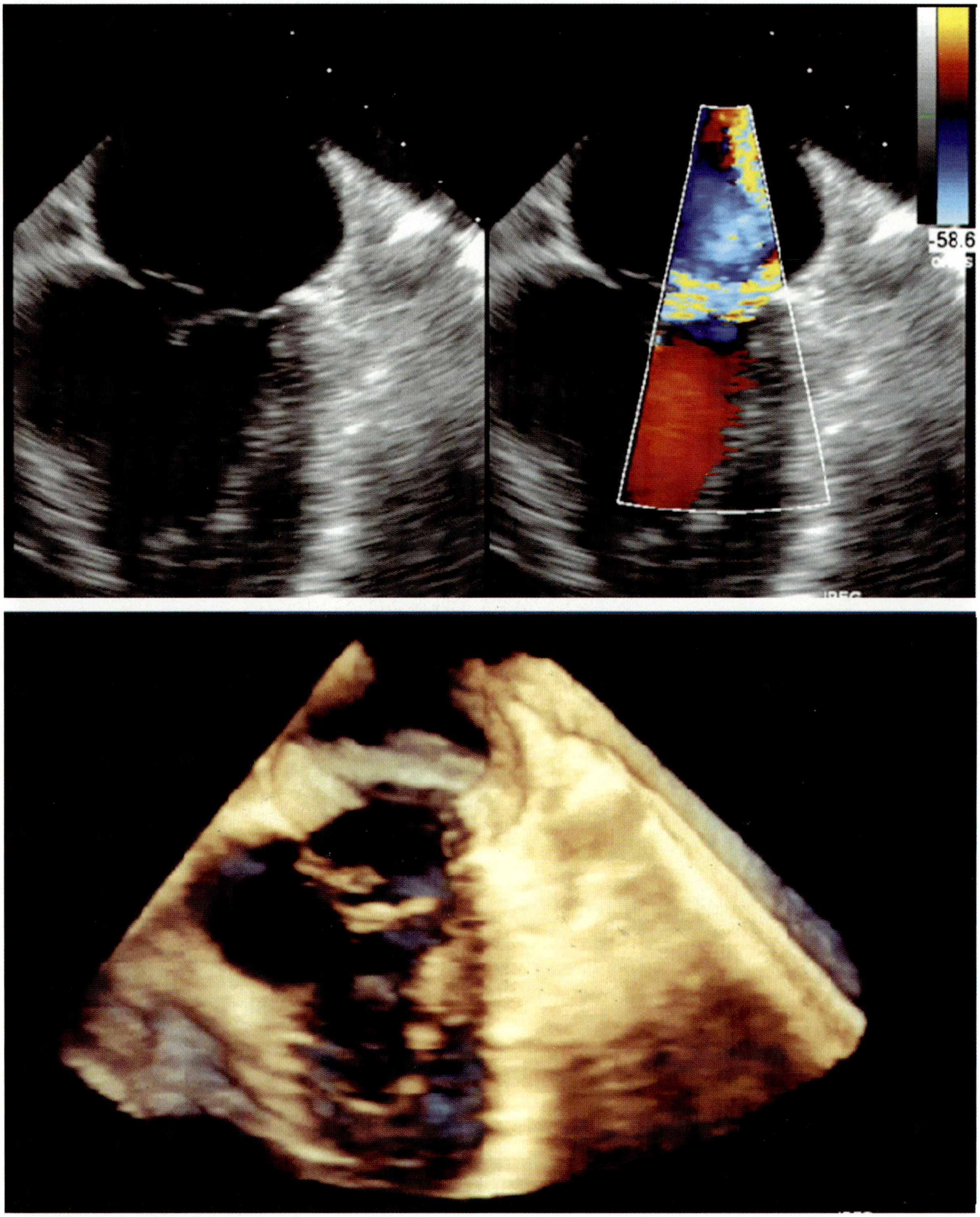

Figure 2: Ischemic MR with submitral aneurysm: The pictures are from a 56-year-old gentleman with coronary artery disease and inferior wall infarction 3 years back with class III symptoms and pan systolic murmur in mitral area. The upper panel showing 2D TEE appearances of 55 degree bicommissural view with color compare view showing grade III mitral regurgitation. The 3D TEE shows clearly the P1,P2 and P3 scallops of Posterior mitral leaflet and the clear documentation of submitral aneurysm

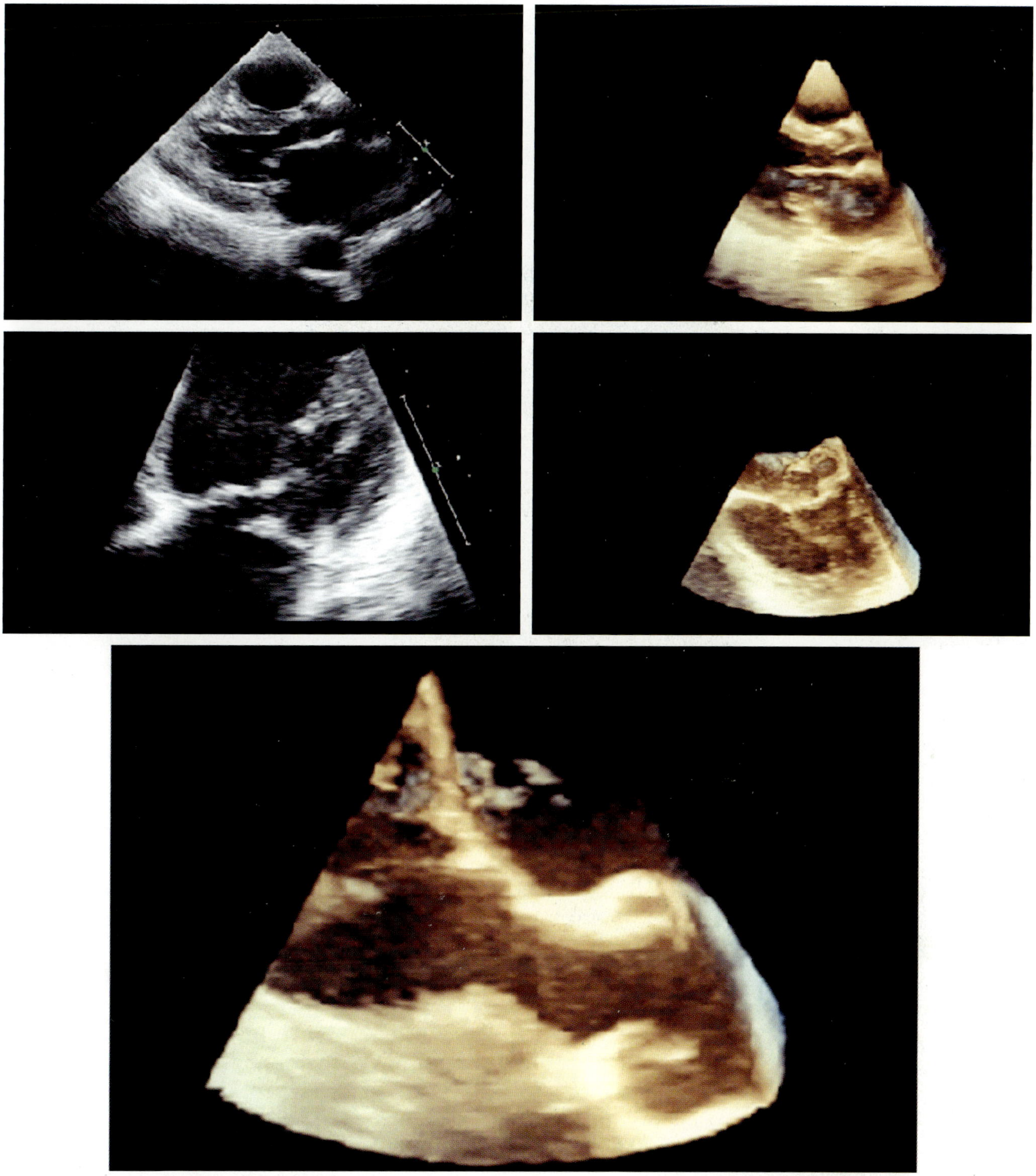

Figure 3: **Flail mitral leaflet with MR:** A 25-year-old young lady admitted with fever and class III dyspnea of 10 days duration and a prominent grade IV pan systolic murmur in mitral area. The transthoracic long axis view in 2D and 3D are shown for direct comparison. The 2D TEE and 3D TEE are shown in the bottom panel. The 3D TEE long axis view shown in the bottom panel clearly shows the vegetation. The clearly flail posterior mitral leaflet is seen in both 3D transthoracic and transesophageal views. The patient had culture positive for *Staph. aureus*

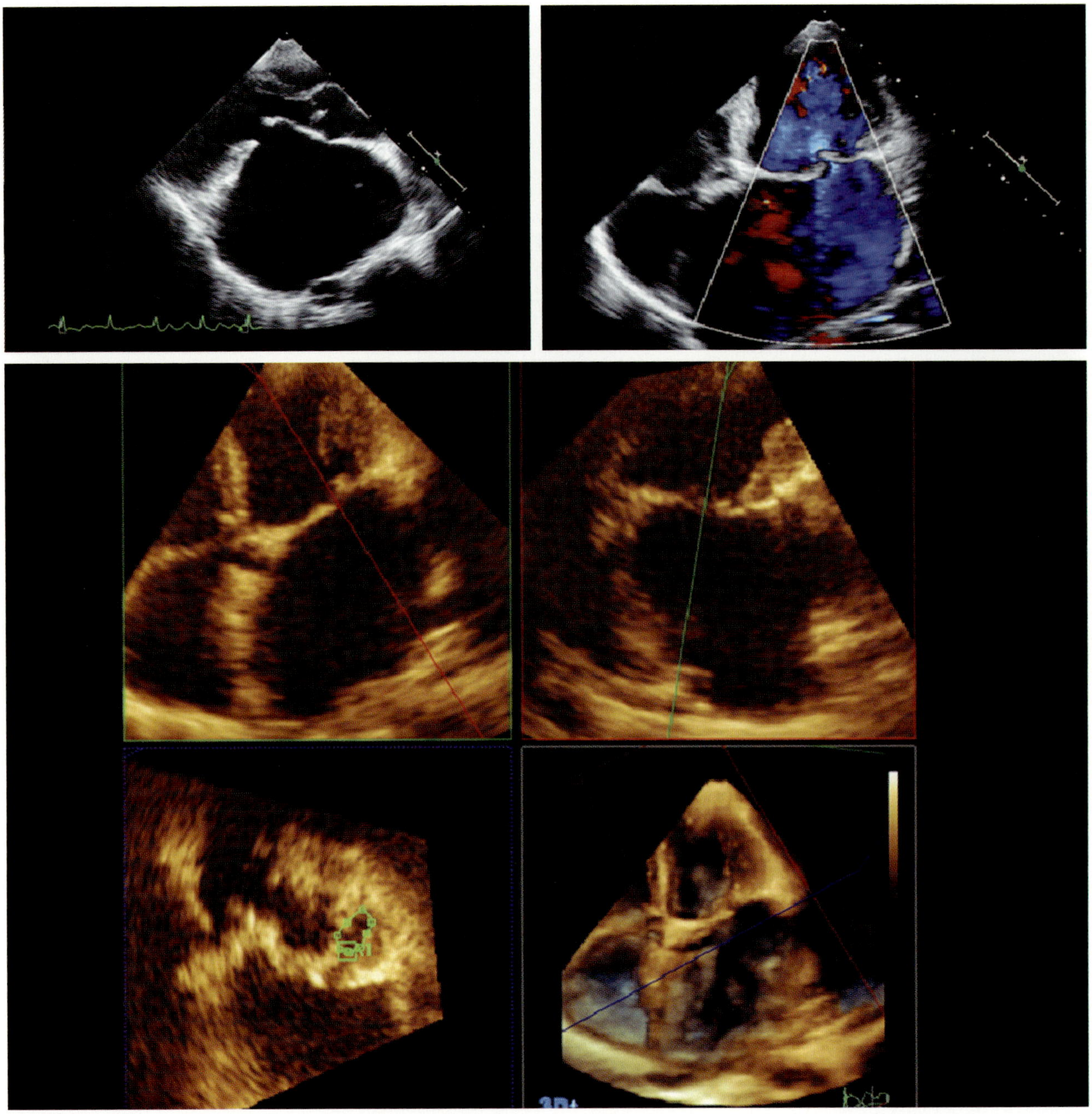

Figure 4: **Rheumatic heart disease with MR:** The sixteen-year-old girl with rheumatic heart disease with severe mitral stenosis (mitral valve area of 0.97 sq.cm) and grade III mitral regurgitation. The markedly thickened mitral valve is seen in all planes with 3D transthoracic echo

QUANTITATIVE 3D ECHOCARDIOGRAPHY

The conventional 2D PISA method assumes a hemispheric shape for PISA. 3DE can address the real geometry and area of the isovelocity surface. 3D color Doppler is indispensable for assessing PISA and MR severity when PISA shape is not hemispheric. 3D color Doppler methods can demonstrate the 3D shape of PISA and allows to correct erroneous calculations of the MR orifice area or regurgitant volume. After acquiring 3D PISA images from a patient with MR, one can check the shape of PISA from multiple views. If it is not a hemisphere, one can change it by lowering aliasing velocities. When the shape of PISA is not a hemisphere, despite the maximal change of the aliasing velocity, more realistic mathematic assumptions such as a curved hemi-ellipsoidal geometry should be applied for determining the PISA area and MR volume. Three-dimensional color Doppler is quite valuable to determine the correctness of using a simple hemispheric PISA method. Quantification of MR can also be done by real time 3D transthoracic echocardiographic measurements of vena contracta area.

FUNCTIONAL AND ISCHEMIC MITRAL REGURGITATION

Understanding the mechanism of Functional Mitral Regurgitation (FMR) requires knowledge about the 3D geometry of the mitral annulus (MA) and the changes that occur during the cardiac cycle. With the advent of 3D Echocardiography, it has become possible to investigate the 3D geometry of the structure with higher accuracy. For the reconstruction of the annulus, the LV volumetric data are segmented into multiple rotational apical planes around the long axis of the annulus using 3D software. Two hinge points of the leaflets (the junction points between the annulus and the leaflets) are then traced in each rotational apical plane. From these data, the 3D image of the annulus is reconstructed by fitting the images and their interpolation together using 3D computer software. On the other hand, using the MPR-guided cropping method, the precise anatomic structures and the anatomic reference points (e.g. Pappillary muscle (PM) head) can be identified separately. The geometric measurements (e.g. distance or angle) between them can then be calculated after placing them on a single plane.

The tethering of both mitral leaflets and their incomplete closure due to the reduced systolic transmitral pressure has been implicated as a main cause of MV deformation in FMR.[13-18] The two papillary muscles have their chordae distributed only to the ipsilateral half portion of the MV leaflets. Therefore, the MV tethering pattern produced by the unilateral PM displacement, which is probably provoked by localized posterior wall remodeling such as lone inferior Myocardial Infarction (MI), is expected to be different from the one that occurs with bilateral PM displacement due to global LV remodeling caused by DCM or ischemic cardiomyopathy with chronic severe LV dysfunction. The combined use of 3D echocardiography and the MPR mode for 3D image analysis may provide more detailed information on its geometry than conventional 2D echocardiography and lead to the development of new strategies for the surgical treatment of FMR.

3D echocardiography has provided important mechanistic insights into functional and ischemic mitral regurgitation resulting from derangements of the normal spatial relationships of the mitral valve leaflets to its chordal attachments, papillary muscles, and the LV (Figures 1 and 2). Distortion of the normal spatial relationship between the LV and mitral valve apparatus results in papillary muscle displacement and tethering of the mitral leaflets, leading to incomplete closure of the leaflets and mitral regurgitation. The 3D echocardiography technique has identified changes in annular shape occurring with functional mitral regurgitation. These mechanistic and anatomic insights based on 3D analysis have provided the basis for the development of new approaches to treating ischemic mitral regurgitation.

MITRAL VALVE PROLAPSE

RT3DE has provided important insight into mitral valve structure, demonstrating the saddle shape of the mitral annulus, with high points located anteriorly and low points oriented in a mediolateral direction. This has helped clarify the appropriate diagnostic imaging planes from which mitral valve prolapse should be diagnosed, thereby avoiding falsepositive interpretations. Accurate determination of a prolapsed leaflet is essential for the successful valve plasty for mitral valve prolapse. MV prolapse can be visualized and quantified with 3DE.[19-25] Such preoperative assessment of the MV morphology is very important to plan the surgical approach (MV repair is preferable to MV replacement).[26] Here 3D has big advantages compared with 2D echocardiography in the communication with the cardiac surgeon describing which scallops are involved or are prolapsing.[27]

FLAIL MITRAL LEAFLET

In patients with mitral regurgitation due to flail leaflet, the lesion results in uniformly high degrees of regurgitation and is reliably diagnosed noninvasively by echocardiography (Figure 3). In Western countries, flail mitral leaflet is the most frequent cause of mitral regurgitation requiring surgical correction. The direction taken by the mitral regurgitation jet provides valuable clues as to the etiology of mitral regurgitation. In general, an eccentric jet suggests an anatomic abnormality resulting in flail or partial flail of one leaflet. The jet direction is opposite to that of the involved leaflet. As such, a posterior flail leaflet generally results in an anteriorly directed jet, whereas the converse is true for an anterior flail leaflet.

Three-dimensional echocardiography provides a detailed anatomic depiction of the mitral valve. In patients with severe mitral regurgitation due to flail mitral valve leaflet, it allows to precisely locate the diseased portion of the leaflets and also in precise quantification of mitral regurgitation.

RHEUMATIC MITRAL REGURGITATION

Rheumatic heart disease is characterized by thickening and sclerosis, primarily of the leaflet tips. The leaflets have a diastolic "hockey stick" appearance or a 90-degree angulation from the chordae to the leaflet tip due to commissural and chordal fusion (Figure 4). Leaflet retraction with incomplete leaflet coaptation is also common. In acute rheumatic fever, focal nodular thickening or discrete small vegetations may be identified. These nodules measure 1 to 5 mm, have a soft tissue echoreflectance, and are located more commonly at the leaflets' coaptation point. In recurrent rheumatic fever, anterior leaflet prolapse may be seen. Unlike infective endocarditis, rheumatic leaflet nodules do not have independent mobility.

CONCLUSION

Because 3DE provides unique tools to assess valves preoperatively, it will play an important role in surgical planning in the future. Valve annulus size, shape, and dynamic changes can be determined accurately, and the patient's individual case can be considered in the treatment by developing and providing customized implants.

Although surgical planning will be one important application of 3DE before treatment, guiding the procedure itself is becoming increasingly important. RT3DE is an ideal tool for offering visual feedback during the procedure, especially with percutaneous interventions.

Because valve pathologies are extremely complex, it is necessary to address the whole valve apparatus, like for the MV, the annulus, the leaflets, the chordae length, and the positioning of the papillary muscles, being influenced by myocardial conditions. 3DE greatly improves the understanding of the interaction of those components and therefore leads to a more complete picture of the pathology and to a more profound choice of treatment.

The ability to reslice a volume offline will transfer a substantial part of the work currently done on the ultrasound system to offline review workstations. Also, physicians from remote places can have access to such a virtual rescan and deliver a second opinion, which makes telemedicine a more realistic scenario rather than just exchanging images and clips.

3DE is a valuable tool to be used in addition to and not instead of 2D echocardiography by providing complementary information and improved quantitative accuracy and reproducibility compared with 2D techniques. By overcoming the current limitations like the lower temporal resolution, compared with 2D echocardiography, 3DE has the potential to become the standard echocardiographic examination procedure for the assessment of valvular disease. The accompanying video (Chapter 4 video 1) illustrates the use of 3D Color Doppler Echocardiography in a patient with Rheumatic Mitral regurgitation and X plane Color Doppler viewing of Mitral Regurgitation (Chapter 4 video 2)

REFERENCES

1. Hung J, Lang R, et al. 3D echocardiography: a review of the current status and future directions. J Am Soc Echocardiogr 2007;20(3):213-33.
2. Nanda N, Sorrell V. Atlas of 3D echocardiography. Valvular heart disease. Armonk (NY): Futura Publishing; 2002. p. 49-94.
3. Valocik G, Kamp O, Visser CA. Three-dimensional echocardiography in mitral valve disease. Eur J Echocardiogr 2005;6(6):443-54.
4. Salehian O, Chan KL. Impact of 3D echocardiography in valvular heart disease. Curr Opin Cardiol 2005;20(2):122-6.
5. Hoda MR, Schwarz T, Wolf I, et al. Three-dimensional echocardiography in cardiac surgery: current status and perspectives. Chirurg 2007;78(5):435-42.
6. Sugeng L, Coon P, Weinert L, et al. Use of real-time 3-dimensional transthoracic echocardiography in the evaluation of mitral valve disease. J Am Soc Echocardiogr 2006;19(4):413-21.

7. Bernhard Mumm, Rolf Baumann, Martin Hyca. Three-Dimensional Echo for the Assessment of Valvular Heart Disease, Cardiol Clin 25 (2007) 283-95.
8. Hozumi T, Yoshikawa J, Yoshida K, et al. Assessment of flail mitral leaflets by dynamic three-dimensional echocardiographic imaging. Am J Cardiol 1997;79:223-5.
9. Chauvel C, Bogino E, Clerc P, et al. Usefulness of three dimensional echocardiography for the evaluation of mitral valve prolapse: an intraoperative study. J Heart Valve Dis 2000;9:341-9.
10. Delabays A, Jeanrenaud X, Chassot PG, et al. Localization and quantification of mitral valve prolapse using three-dimensional echocardiography. Eur J Echocardiogr 2004;5:422-9.
11. Macnab A, Jenkins NP, Bridgewater BJ, et al. Three dimensional echocardiography is superior to multiplane transoesophageal echo in the assessment of regurgitant mitral valve morphology. Eur J Echocardiogr 2004;5:212-22.
12. Ryan LP, Salgo IS, Gorman RC, et al. The emerging role of three-dimensional echocardiography in mitral valve repair. Semin Thorac Cardiovasc Surg 2006;18:126-34.
13. He S, Fontaine AA, Schwammenthal E, et al. Integrated mechanism for functional mitral regurgitation: leaflet restriction versus coapting force: in vitro studies. Circulation 1997;96:1826-34.
14. Otsuji Y, Handschumacher MD, Schwammenthal E, et al. Insights from three-dimensional echocardiography into the mechanism of functional mitral regurgitation: direct in vivo demonstration of altered leaflet tethering geometry. Circulation 1997;96:1999-2008.
15. Otsuji Y, Handschumacher MD, Liel-Cohen N, et al. Mechanism of ischemic mitral regurgitation with segmental left ventricular dysfunction: three-dimensional echocardiographic studies in models of acute and chronic progressive regurgitation. J Am Coll Cardiol 2001;37:641-8.
16. Kwan J, Shiota T, Agler DA, et al. Geometric differences of the mitral apparatus between ischemic and dilated cardiomyopathy with significant mitral regurgitation: real-time three-dimensional echocardiography study. Circulation 2003; 107:1135-40.
17. Song JM, Qin JX, Kongsaerepong V, et al. Determinants of ischemic mitral regurgitation in patients with chronic anterior wall myocardial infarction: a real time three dimensional echocardiography study. Echocardiography 2006;23:650-7.
18. Watanabe N, Ogasawara Y, Yamaura Y, et al. Quantitation of mitral valve tenting in ischemic mitral regurgitation by transthoracic real-time three-dimensional echocardiography. J Am Coll Cardiol 2005;45:763-9.
19. Chauvel C, Bogino E, Clerc P, et al. Usefulness of 3D echocardiography for the evaluation of mitral valve prolapse: an intraoperative study. J Heart Valve Dis 2000;9(3):341-9.
20. Levine RA, Handschumacher MD, Sanfilippo AJ, et al. Three-dimensional echocardiographic reconstruction of the mitral valve, with implications for the diagnosis of mitral valve prolapse. Circulation 1989;80(3):589-98.
21. Chung R, Pepper J, Henein M. Images in cardiology: mitral valve anterior leaflet prolapse by real- time 3D transthoracic echocardiography. Heart (British Cardiac Society) 2005;91(9): e55.
22. Pepi M, Tamborini G, Maltagliati A, et al. Head-to-head comparison of 2- and 3D transthoracic and transesophageal echocardiography in the localization of mitral valve prolapse. J Am Coll Cardiol 2006;48(12):2524-30.
23. Delabays A, Jeanrenaud X, Chassot PG, et al. Localization and quantification of mitral valve prolapse using 3D echocardiography. Eur J Echocardiogr 2004;5(6):422-9.
24. Patel V, Hsiung MC, Nanda NC, et al. Usefulness of live/real time 3D transthoracic echocardiography in the identification of individual segment/scallop prolapsed of the mitral valve. Echocardiography 2006; 23(6):513-8.
25. Müller S, Bartel T. Comparison of 3D imaging to transesophageal echocardiography for preoperative evaluation in mitral valve prolapse. Am J Cardiol 2006;98:243-8.
26. Galloway AC, Colvin SB, Baumann FG, et al. A comparison of mitral valve reconstruction with mitral valve replacement: intermediate-term results. Ann Thorac Surg 1989;47(5):655-62.
27. Ahmed S, Nanda NC, Miller AP, et al. Usefulness of transesophageal 3D echocardiography in the identification of individual segment/scallop prolapse of the mitral valve. Echocardiography 2003;20(2):203-9.

CHAPTER 5

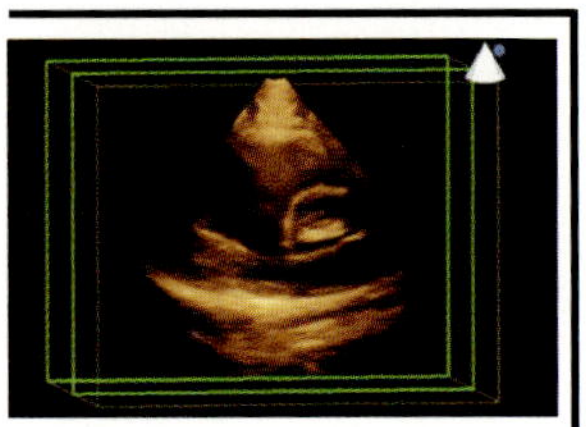

Three-Dimensional Echocardiography in Aortic and Tricuspid Valve Disease

V Amuthan, A Jegadeeswari

AORTIC VALVE DISEASE

Three-dimensional echocardiography has been applied for anatomic assessment of the aortic valve and root morphology and to calculate the valve area in aortic stenosis. The technique has been used to delineate aortic flow patterns and has demonstrated feasibility and accuracy in quantifying aortic regurgitation. Other applications have included the detection and localization of aortic valve vegetations, assessment of congenital outflow obstruction abnormalities, and demonstration of morphological changes in the valve after balloon dilation.

To examine the aortic valve with RT3DE, a high right or left parasternal approach gives the best results. The apical window is another option but has the aortic valve (AoV) positioned in the far field. For a complete valvular assessment, the aortic valve becomes more and more important. Studies have shown that 3DE improves the morphological assessment of the AoV leaflets, the quantification of the valve orifice area in aortic stenosis, and the quantification of aortic regurgitation (Figures 1A to F). The accompanying video (Chapter 5 video 1) shows Live 3D Echocardiographic view of a case of Bicuspid Aortic valve with above downward orientation of cusps and mild Aortic Stenosis. Video 2 shows the short axis view of Aortic root abscess in a patient with Infective endocarditis Video 3 shows the 3D Trans Esophageal Echocardiographic view of a normal trileaflet Aortic valve.

BIPLANE AND FULL-VOLUME THREE-DIMENSIONAL ECHOCARDIOGRAPHY

Full-volume 3D echocardiography can provide a pyramidal image of the whole heart and the volume rendered image can be rotated and observed from any direction. The aortic valve can be observed from the direction of the ascending aorta, which is impossible by 2D echocardiography. Aortic annular motion affects the calculation of AVA using 2DTEE. Volumetric 3DTEE data sets encompass the entire AV, and thus, allow the delineation of the tangential 2D cut plane at the tip of the AV cusps. Two-dimensional planimetric calculation of AVA from volumetric 3D TEE data sets is a new useful technique for measuring anatomical AVA in patients with AS. Three-dimensional transesophageal echocardiography has a potential for more accurate determination of anatomical AVA. Although 3D TEE monitoring is not a standard procedure during PAVR, when used in combination with conventional 2D TEE, it contributes to improving adequate patient selection and provides more accurate information to the interventional cardiologist during positioning, deployment, and early function of the prosthesis during transcatheter aortic valve replacement.

THREE-DIMENSIONAL COLOR DOPPLER ECHOCARDIOGRAPHY

Three-dimensional color Doppler facilitates morphologic assessment of the flow jet and helps to appreciate the 3D vena contracta with acceleration flow. The regurgitant orifice is often an elliptic or irregular oval, which changes the width of the vena contracta in different views. 3D color Doppler echocardiography is a useful tool in the visualization of the actual shape of the regurgitant orifice. 3D color flow VC area measurement provides a simple and accurate method for assessing the severity of AR.

PITFALLS IN THE ASSESSMENT OF THE AORTIC VALVE BY REAL-TIME 3D ECHO

Thus 3D echocardiography can provide additional anatomic information compared to 2D echocardiography. However,

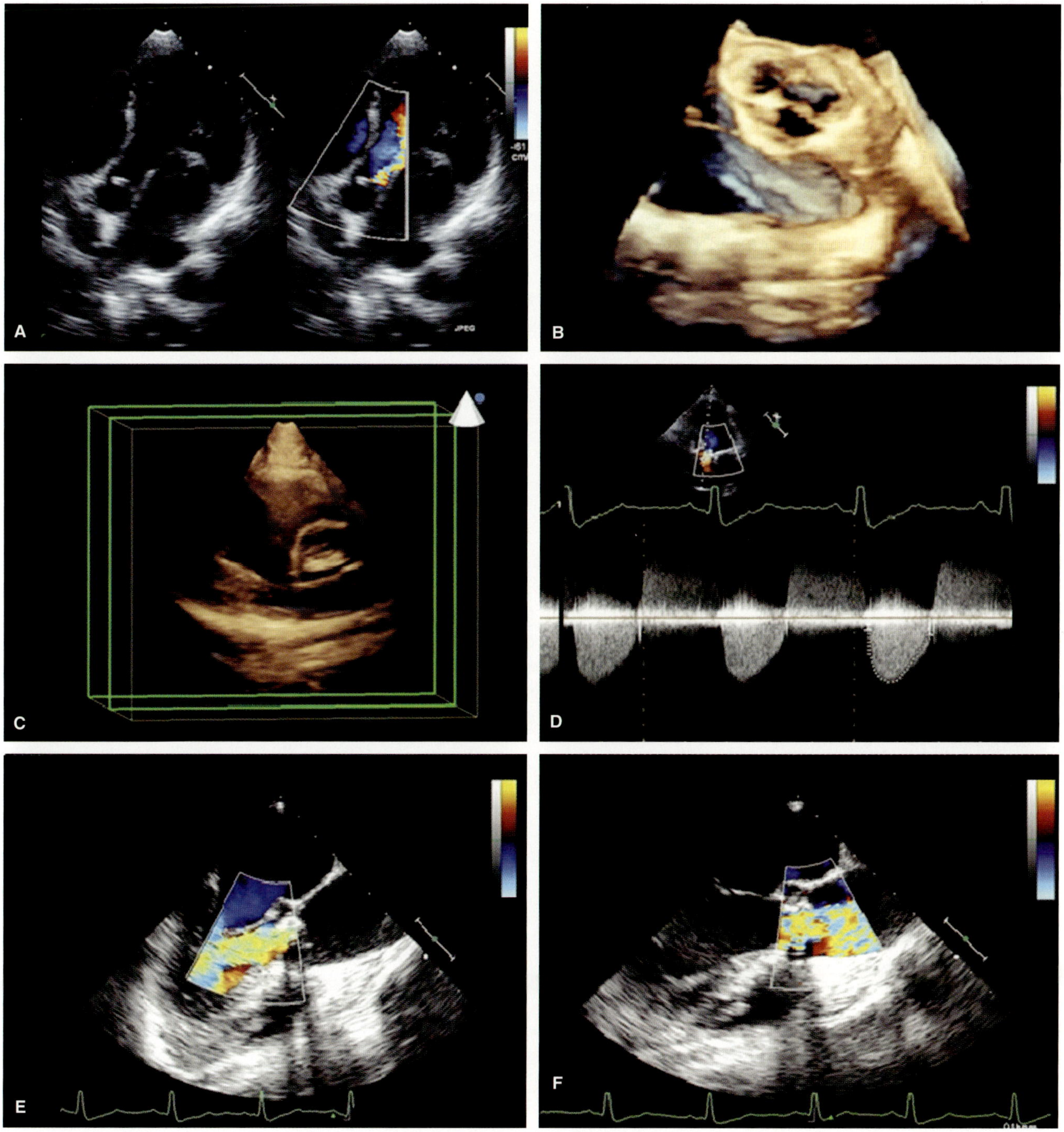

Figures 1A to F: Echo imaging of aortic valve: (A) Apical long axis in a patient with RHD, mitral stenosis and aortic stenosis and AR. (B) 3D TEE showing the thickened trileaflet aortic valve with remarkable thickening. (C) 3D Echo in a patient with calcific aortic valve seen in short axis plane. (D) Spectral Doppler echocardiogram showing a peak gradient of 73 mm of Hg and mean gradient of 44 mm of Hg. (E) Showing the grade IV aortic regurgitation jet. (F) Showing the aortic stenotic jet

limitations of 3DE for assessing the aortic valve are the temporal resolution of 3DE. Because of the relatively poor image quality in current real-time 3D echocardiography the 3D image alone is not sufficient to make a diagnosis.

TRICUSPID VALVE

Compared with the MV and AoV, much less work has been published to study the tricuspid valve (TV) and pulmonary valve (PV) with 3DE techniques. In order to acquire a

RT3DE data set of the TV, it is recommended to use more gain than normal while positioning the RT3DE transducer in a modified parasternal long axis position, centering the TV in the 3D volume. From an apical four-chamber view, the TV can be visualized in relation to other intracardiac structures. Thus, RT3DE allows the visualization of all three TV leaflets, their attachment in the TV annulus, and their relation with the interventricular septum. 3DE also can provide an accurate visualization of the TV from a surgical viewpoint from the right atrium to help in the surgical decision-making process. In standard two-dimensional (2D) echocardiography, it is difficult to visualize all three leaflets in one view whereas all three leaflets of the tricuspid valve are clearly visualized in the 3D images seen from the right ventricle.

TRICUSPID REGURGITATION AND GEOMETRY OF THE TRICUSPID VALVE

Tricuspid annular dilatation and tethering of the leaflets of the tricuspid valve are important changes in the tricuspid valve geometry in patients with functional tricuspid regurgitation. Tricuspid annuloplasty is recommended for the treatment of functional tricuspid regurgitation as a standard surgical procedure at the time of left-sided heart surgery to decrease the postoperative morbidity and mortality because of significant tricuspid regurgitation. Although an annuloplasty ring is commonly used in this surgical procedure, residual tricuspid regurgitation commonly occurs. One major reason for this unsatisfactory result may be inadequate knowledge of the three-dimensional (3D) geometry of the tricuspid valve. The 3D geometry of the tricuspid valve can be analyzed with custom-made software for the analysis of 3D echocardiographic data obtained from real-time 3D echocardiography. To acquire the 3D geometry of the tricuspid annulus, the location of eight annulus points should be pinpointed throughout a cardiac cycle from four cross-sectional planes rotated at 450 about a fixed rotational axis. Studies have shown that the more severe the tricuspid regurgitation, the more planar the tricuspid annulus. This is to be considered in tricuspid annuloplasty in patients with tricuspid regurgitation.

BIBLIOGRAPHY

1. Bernhard Mumm, Rolf Baumann, Martin Hyca, Three-Dimensional Echo for the Assessment of Valvular Heart Disease, Cardiol Clin 25 (2007) 283-95.
2. Goland S, Trento A, Iida K, et al: Assessment of aortic stenosis by three dimensional echocardiography: an accurate and novel approach. Heart 2007;93:801-7.
3. Gutierrez-Chico JL, Zamorano JL, Prieto-Moriche E, et al: Real-time three-dimensional echocardiography in aortic stenosis: a novel, simple, and reliable method to improve accuracy in area calculation. Eur Heart J 2008;29:1296-1306.
4. Handke M, Jahnke C, Heinrichs G, et al. New 3D echocardiographic system using digital radiofrequency data-visualization and quantitative analysis of aortic valve dynamics with high resolution: methods, feasibility, and initial clinical experience. Circulation 2003;107(23):2876-9.
5. Hoda MR, Schwarz T, Wolf I, et al. Three-dimensional echocardiography in cardiac surgery: current status and perspectives. Chirurg 2007;78(5):435-42.
6. Hung J, Lang R, et al. 3D echocardiography: a review of the current status and future directions. J Am Soc Echocardiogr 2007;20(3):213-33.
7. Masaki N, Guerra V, Roman KS, et al. Three-dimensional tricuspid annular function provides insight into the mechanism of tricuspid valve regurgitation in classic hypoplastic left heart syndrome. J Am Soc Echocardiogr 2006;19(4):391-402.
8. Nanda N, Sorrell V. Atlas of 3D echocardiography. Valvular heart disease. Armonk (NY): Futura Publishing; 2002; pp. 49-94.
9. Salehian O, Chan KL. Impact of 3D echocardiography in valvular heart disease. Curr Opin Cardiol 2005;20(2):122-6.
10. Sugeng L, Shernan SK, Lang R, et al. Real-time 3D transesophageal echocardiographic assessment of cardiac structures. J Am Soc Echocardiogr 2007;20(5):570.

CHAPTER 6

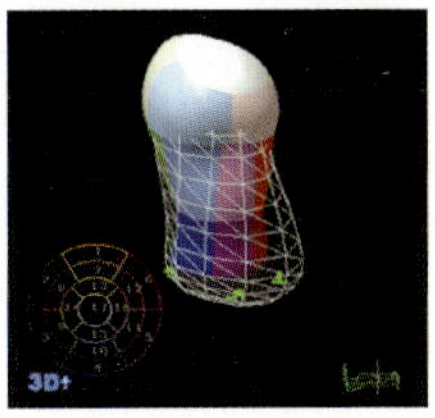

Three-Dimensional Echocardiography in Coronary Artery Disease

V Amuthan, R Aravazhi

INTRODUCTION

The advancement in the 3D evaluation in coronary artery disease is enormous and more and more uses are being described every day in the recent publications. However, 3D Echocardiography is particularly useful in following situations:

1. Evaluation of heart chambers: Size, function, and mass
2. Stress echocardiography
3. Complications of myocardial infarction
4. Perfusion assessment.
5. Serial diagnosis of LV systolic asynchrony as a guide for resynchronization therapy.

EVALUATION OF HEART CHAMBERS: SIZE, FUNCTION AND MASS

Volumetric measurements using 3-dimensional echocardiography (3DE) avoid the need for geometric assumptions and the risk of underestimating volumes in foreshortened views. Consequently, the evaluation of left ventricular (LV) volumes and the ejection fraction (EF) has been shown to be more reproducible and accurate with 3DE than both 2-dimensional and M-mode based techniques, when compared with cardiac magnetic resonance (CMR).[1-6] The superiority of the 3DE imaging in terms of improved accuracy[7-12] and reproducibility[12,13] was recently also demonstrated for real-time 3-dimensional echocardiographic (RT3DE) imaging, which allows fast and largely automated volumetric analysis of LV volume and function based on endocardial surface detection.[14]

Over the past decade, a different approach has been pursued to eliminate the need for tedious multiplane acquisition and time-consuming 3D reconstruction altogether. This approach is based on real-time volumetric imaging, which uses transducers containing arrays of piezoelectric elements capable of scanning pyramidal volumes, rather than the conventional 2D phased-array transducers that scan a fan-shaped sector in a single plane. Importantly, real-time volumetric imaging allowed fast acquisition of pyramidal datasets during a single breath-hold without the need for off-line reconstruction, thus eliminating motion artifacts known to have adversely affected the image quality (Figure 1).

One of the main reasons for requesting an echocardiogram in routine clinical practice is the assessment of global and regional LV function. To date, this assessment is predominantly performed using visual interpretation or "eye-balling" of dynamic ultrasound images of the beating heart, which requires adequate training and experience to accurately estimate LVEF and evaluate wall motion. However, the limitations of this subjective interpretation have been long recognized, and consequently the use of quantitative techniques has been recommended. Thus, multiple methods of measuring LV size and function have been developed, validated, and refined for both M-mode and 2D B-mode images, and subsequently for reconstructed 3D images and more recently for volumetric real-time 3D data sets. The relative inaccuracy of the 1-dimensional and 2D echocardiographic approaches has been attributed to the need for geometric modeling of the ventricle. The "missing dimensions" have also been consistently referred

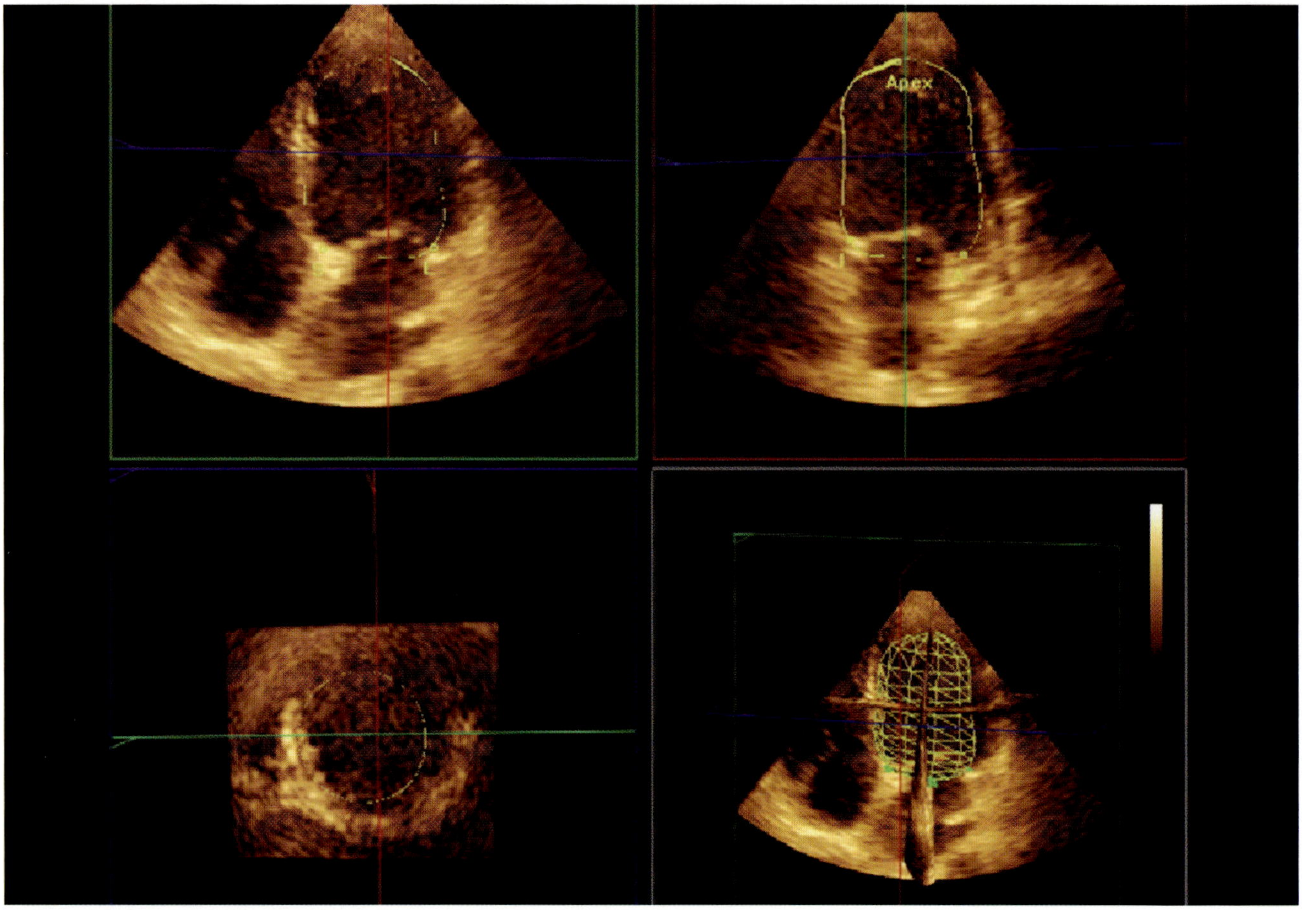

Figure 1: Calculation of left ventricular volume

The following steps are undertaken: The color, brightness, gain and magnify controls are used if necessary to ensure best image clarity. The play or space bar are pressed for a moving image.

In the Blue Quad (Lower Left)

- Move pointer to the intersection of the green and red lines until a "+" appears, and place this point into the center of the LV cavity. Pick up the end of the green line and rotate the green plane until a true four-chamber view is seen in the green quad (upper left).
- Position the yellow arrow so that it intersects the midpoint of the ventricular septum.
- Press pause or space bar to **freeze** the image and ensure you are on **end diastolic frame**. This will be frame one if ECG triggering was used to acquire image.

In the Green Quad (Upper Left)

- Pick up the end of the red line and rotate the red plane while looking at the red quad (Upper right) to ensure the LV is not foreshortened.

In the Red Quad

- Pick up the end of the green line and rotate the green plane looking at the green quad to ensure the LV is not foreshortened.

to as the main source of the relatively wide inter-measurement variability of the echocardiographic estimates of ventricular size and function. In addition, the frequently encountered limitations in endocardial visualization, particularly in the apical-lateral segments of the LV, are commonly compensated for by tilting the transducer. This maneuver generally improves endocardial visualization, but at the same time generates oblique or foreshortened views of the ventricle, resulting in even less accurate and reproducible measurements. In this regard, the biggest advantage of 3D echocardiography is the lack of dependence on geometric modeling and image plane positioning, which theoretically should result in accurate chamber quantification (Figure 2).[15] The accompanying video (Chapter 6 video 1) shows the assessment of 3D Left ventricular function in a patient with Coronary Artery disease.

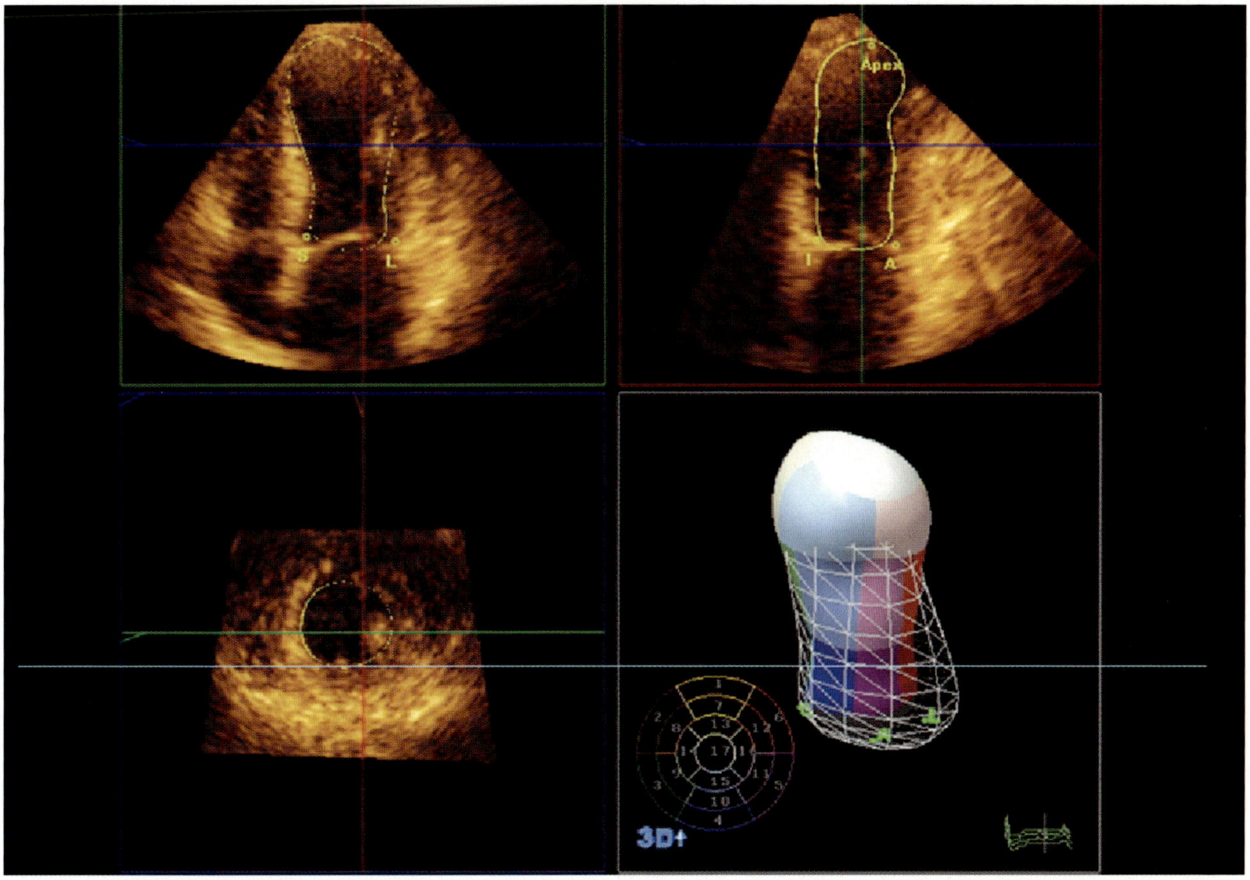

Figure 2: How to perform the analysis

- Go to the top of the tools menu (top left screen) and click on **End Diastolic Volume**.
- **Place five points in this order** onto the images in the upper quads: septum, basal, anterior, inferior, apical. The first four basal points should be placed at the base of the walls just within the tissue. The apical point can be placed in either quad.
- ***The end diastolic volume will then be calculated and displayed top right of screen.***
- If it is necessary to edit the border: Select **add ref points** (top left). Click on image where the border should be. Select update to re-compute volume and finish to continue.
- Choose the end systolic frame along the yellow bar. In the tools menu, click on **end systolic volume**. Repeat steps to place the five points. The end systolic volume will be displayed with the EF. Add reference points as before if editing of border is necessary.
- Select **Sequence Analysis** on the tools menu to initiate the software to track the endocardial border in every frame in the loop. This takes a few moments to complete.
- **Editing** can be performed in any frame if necessary. Select **start edit** and click on image where you think the border should be and **Finish edit** to complete. Select **show report page** to display volume curves and synchronicity information.
- The Figure 2 shown above illustrates a patient with anterior wall myocardial infarction with left ventricular apical aneurysm with all segments displayed in the lower right quad in both the bull's eye plot and in the segmental mode.

Nevertheless, almost all studies that have directly compared the accuracy of 3D measurements of LV volumes and Ejection Fraction have shown the superiority of the 3D approach over the 2D methodology, which was shown to consistently underestimate LV volumes. This superiority was shown in both accuracy and reproducibility when compared against independent reference techniques, such as radionuclide ventriculography or magnetic resonance imaging (MRI).[16-18] Although in earlier 3D studies, quantification of LV size and function relied on tedious, manual, or at best semi-automated tracing of endocardial boundaries in multiple planes, today it is based on near fully automated frame-by-frame detection of the 3D endocardial surface as several studies have reported significant improvements in the accuracy and reproducibility of 3D estimates of LV mass compared with their traditional M-mode and 2D counterparts.

Similar results confirming improved accuracy and reproducibility of the 3D approach were reported by investigators who compared 2D and 3D echocardiographic measurements of left and right atrial volumes against an independent gold standard.[19,20] These findings may have important clinical implications on the diagnosis and management of patients with atrial fibrillation, diastolic dysfunction, and acute myocardial infarction.

Because of its complex geometrical crescent shape, the estimation of right ventricular volumes based on geometric modeling from 2D images has been extremely challenging. Thus, not surprisingly, the intrinsic ability of 3D imaging to directly measure right ventricular volumes without the need for geometrical modeling has resulted in significant improvements in accuracy and reproducibility compared with previously used 2D techniques[21-23] (Figure 3).

Diagnosis of regional wall motion abnormalities in echocardiographic studies is routinely performed by visually integrating regional endocardial motion and wall thickness. The reproducibility of this interpretation is limited because of its subjective nature, which is also extremely dependent on the experience of the reader. This is of particular concern in patients with suboptimal image quality that impedes endocardial visualization. Not only may endocardial segments that are poorly visualized be incorrectly interpreted as having abnormal wall motion, but also discrete areas of hypokinesis may be missed because they are simply not visualized in the standard imaging planes. It is not uncommon for an echocardiographer performing the test to slightly change transducer orientation to "better see" a specific myocardial segment. Such maneuvers can make a myocardial segment look like an area of hypokinesis, or alternatively, can make an apparent wall motion abnormality disappear, and thus affect the diagnostic accuracy of the test. In this regard, volumetric imaging is different because the 3D data set contains the complete dynamic information on LV chamber contraction and filling.

STRESS ECHO

Main limitations for conventional 2D stress echocardiography are problems during acquisition on one hand and of data analysis on the other hand. Data acquisition may be impaired by:

- Probe positioning errors resulting in inadequate image planes
- A reduced image quality during transthoracic scanning with poor visualization of left ventricular (LV) walls
- The time-consuming serial acquisition of different image planes–the set of different 2D cut planes (parasternal short and long axis, apical four and two-chamber view as well as apical long axis) has to be acquired in a narrow time window during peak stress while wall motion abnormalities exist.

Importantly, 3D data sets are acquired virtually instantaneously, and any 2D view can be obtained from them simply by cropping out or "peeling off" the rest of the information. In addition, the function of any ventricular wall can be objectively assessed by measuring a variety of wall motion parameters.[24] For these reasons, 3D data sets are extremely appealing for the evaluation of regional LV function. Real-time 3D imaging has been recently used during dobutamine stress testing and found to be feasible and useful for the detection of stress-induced wall motion abnormalities.[25,26] Several other studies have explored the potential of quantitative evaluation of regional LV function based on segmental analysis of the dynamic 3D endocardial surface.[24]

Like conventional 2D techniques, 3D echo during the stress echo workflow then is performed at rest, at low and peak stress, and during recovery. Both physical stress (either bicycle or treadmill exercise) and pharmacological stress (mainly dobutamine plus atropine) have been used in combination with 3D techniques. Left heart contrast agents can be applied for better endocardial delineation.

Once the 3D data set is acquired, image planes can be created in every desired orientation. Besides the extraction of conventional two-, three- and four-chamber-views, multiple parallel short axis slices can be used for systematic analysis of regional wall motion analysis (Figure 4). These slices can be extracted manually or semi-automatically, as it is meanwhile possible in several commercially available 3D echo machines. The last step of stress echo analysis is a side-by-side analysis of the extracted image planes at different stress/exercise levels still is based on subjective interpretation of wall motion abnormalities. Other viewing options include the slice plane view which shows a beating LV surface mesh within the three orthogonal axis planes and "Show Reference Mesh" which retains an end-diastolic surface mesh against which subsequent wall motion may be compared.

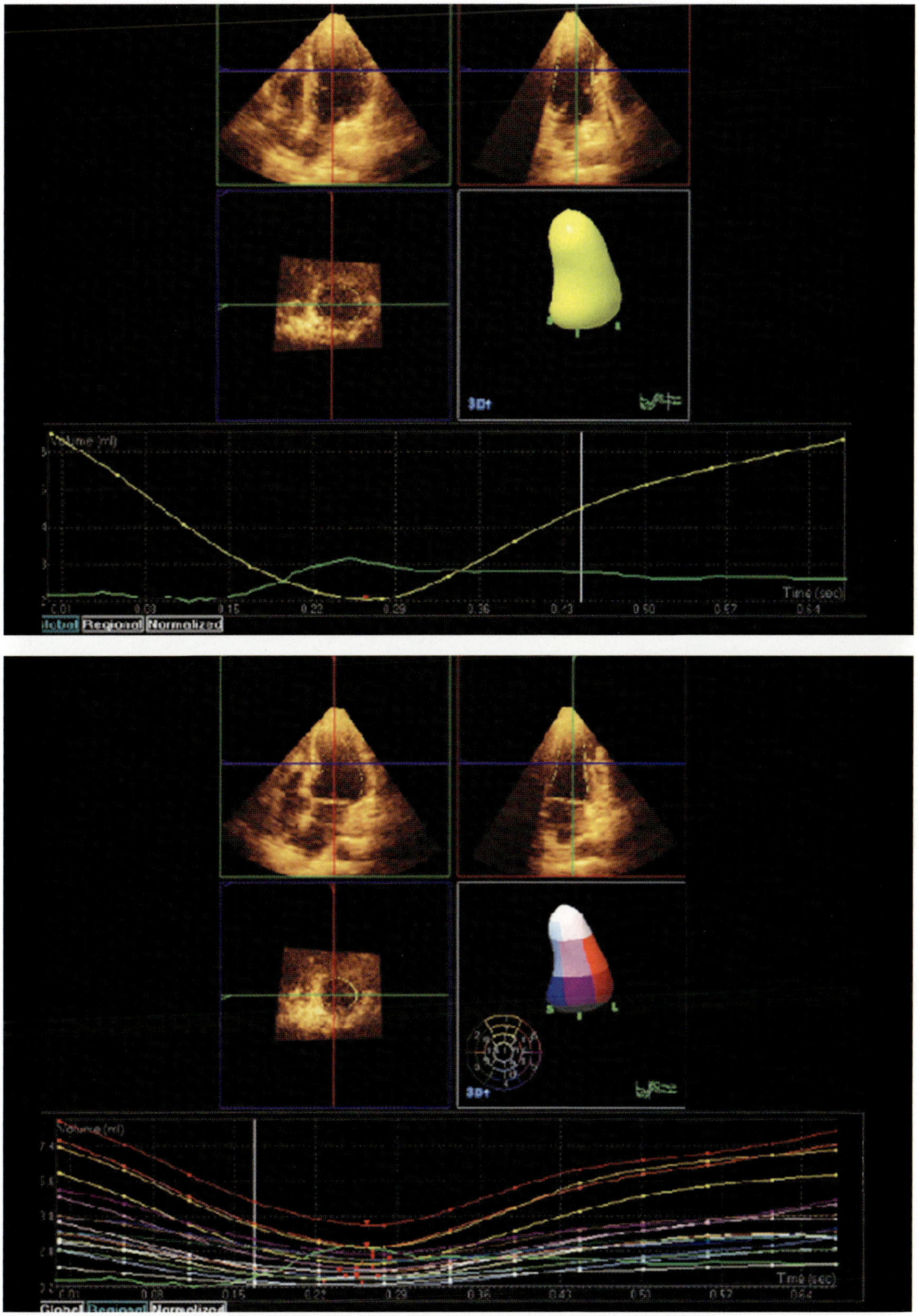

Figure 3: Time volume curve: One of the important indices of regional left ventricular function. The upper panel depicts the global and the lower panel depicts the regional time volume curves

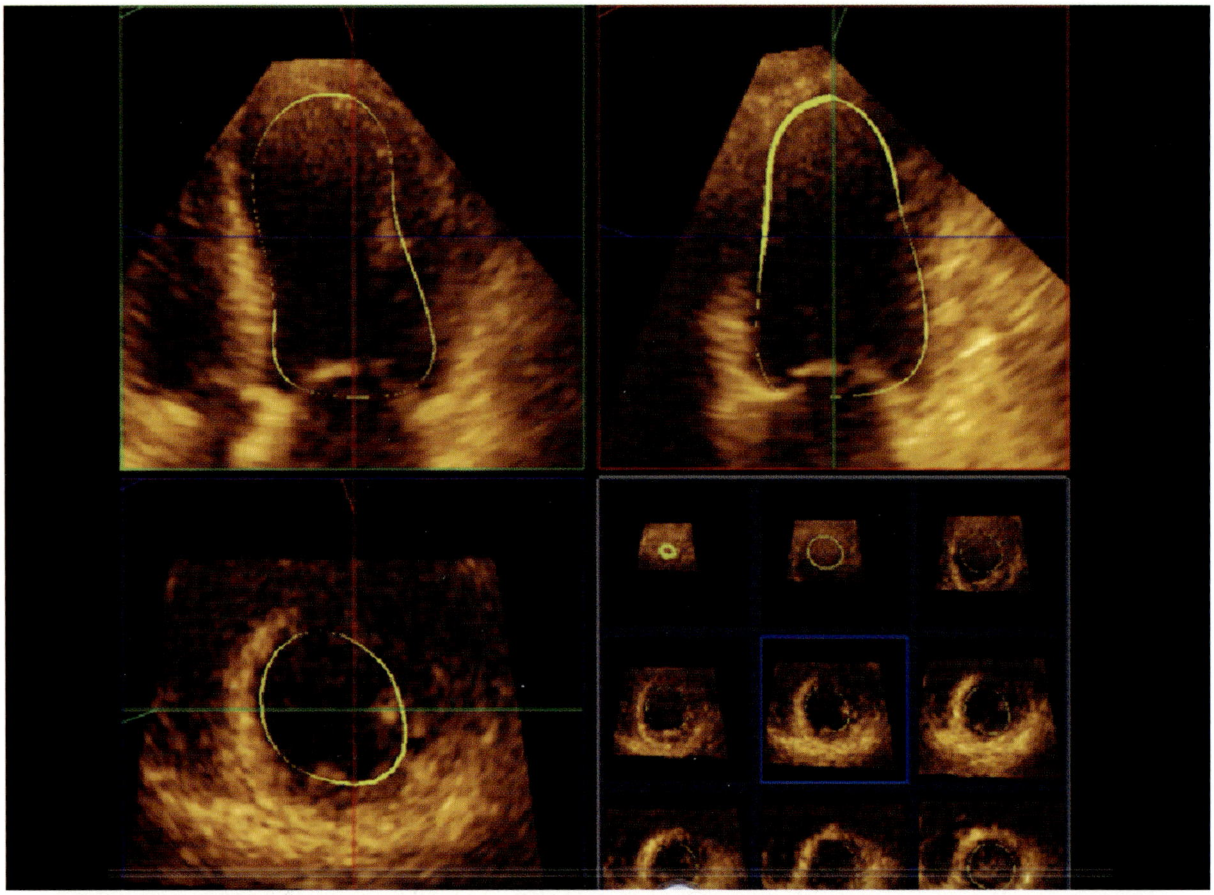

Figure 4: Slice displaying nine serial sections in stress Echo

COMPLICATIONS OF MYOCARDIAL INFARCTION: ISCHEMIC MITRAL REGURGITATION

Ischemic mitral regurgitation (MR) is functional MR caused by coronary artery disease, in particular, right and left circumflex artery disease. The prognostic implication of ischemic MR in the chronic phase is associated with excess mortality independent of baseline characteristics and degree of ventricular function. Possibility for more direct assessment of regurgitant flow volumes and regurgitant orifice using 3D color flow imaging. 3D color Doppler more accurately represents the true shape of the vena contracta (Figure 5).[27] 3D echo may be used to estimate stroke volume and cardiac output and thereby provide better quantification of the severity of regurgitant lesions.[28,29] With the recent advances in 3D imaging techniques, determining the geometric changes of the mitral apparatus that are accompanied by distortion of the regional or global LV chamber have been explored.[30] In these studies, leaflet tethering due to displacement of the papillary muscle has been reported as a main mechanism of functional MR.

LV CLOT

Layered clot in LV apex poses great challenge for diagnosis. Our department series of cases proved superiority of 3D Echo over 2D in early diagnosis of LV apical clot (Figure 6A).

SUBMITRAL ANEURYSM

3D imaging clearly demonstrates position of submitral aneurysm in post-myocardial infarction patients. It also shows effect on mitral valve apparatus (Figure 6B).

VENTRICULAR SEPTAL RUPTURE

Site of ventricular septal rupture is well demonstrated by cropping LV (Figure 6C) .

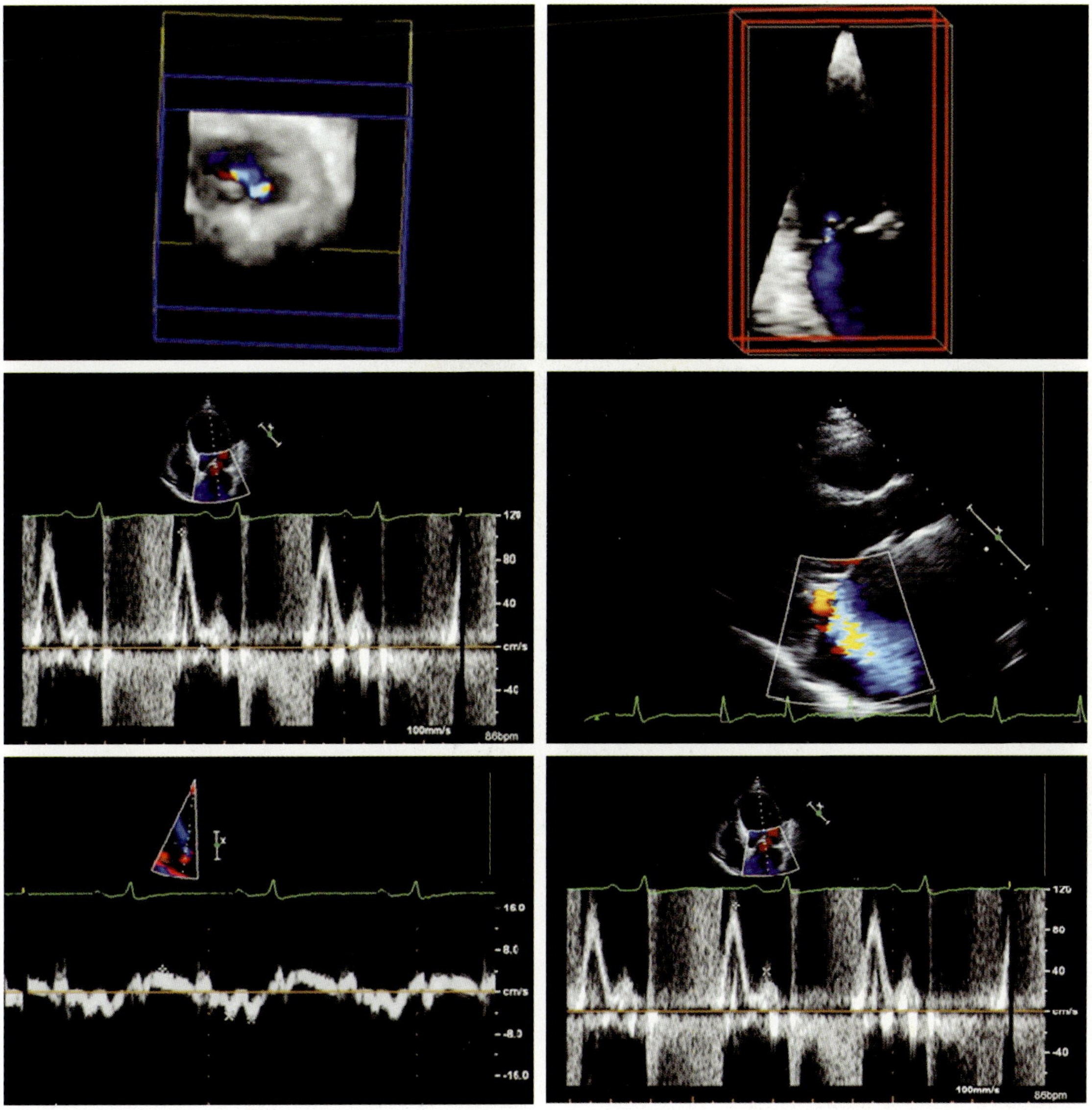

Figure 5: Ischemic mitral regurgitation is shown in the 3D color mode. The venae contracti can be exactly quantified and 3D color is the best way to assess the severity of mitral regurgitation. The top two quads show the 3D MR in two different planes. The middle left quad depicts the pulse wave Doppler mode and the middle right quad showing the 2D color mode. The assessment of the diastolic function also adds another dimension. The E wave deceleration time of 108 msec and the E/A ratio of < 1 signifies restrictive abnormality along with E/E' value of 23 indicates a pulmonary capillary wedge pressure of > 20 mm of Hg

PERFUSION ASSESSMENT

The feasibility of applying volumetric analysis to contrast-enhanced real-time 3D data sets obtained in patients with suboptimal image quality was recently tested. This approach allows quantification of global[31] as well as regional[32] LV function when used with selective dual triggering at end systole and end diastole to reduce the destructive effects of ultrasound on contrast microbubbles. Before the development of real-time 3D imaging, assessment of myocardial perfusion had to remain limited to either visualization of perfusion defects or at best quantification of their size. Quantification of tissue blood flow would require repeated contrast maneuvers, such as bolus injections, which are necessary to assess flow dynamics for each imaging plane, rendering this methodology clinically inapplicable. In contrast, real-time 3D echocardiography offers an opportunity for online volumetric imaging of the entire heart during a single contrast enhancement maneuver. This approach uses continuous infusion of contrast and thus allows ample time to optimize imaging settings. It does not require microbubble destruction by high-energy pulses, but instead uses a brief infusion interruption, which effectively results in a "negative bolus" of contrast.

Another important recent technological development was the incorporation of harmonic imaging and later power modulation imaging[33] into real-time 3D imaging. Despite the lower spatial resolution, these contrast-targeted modes resulted in incremental improvements in the ability to visualize intramyocardial contrast. The lower temporal resolution, which is an intrinsic property of the multipulse power modulation technique, is not a real limitation in the context of perfusion imaging since only one frame per cardiac cycle is required for perfusion analysis.

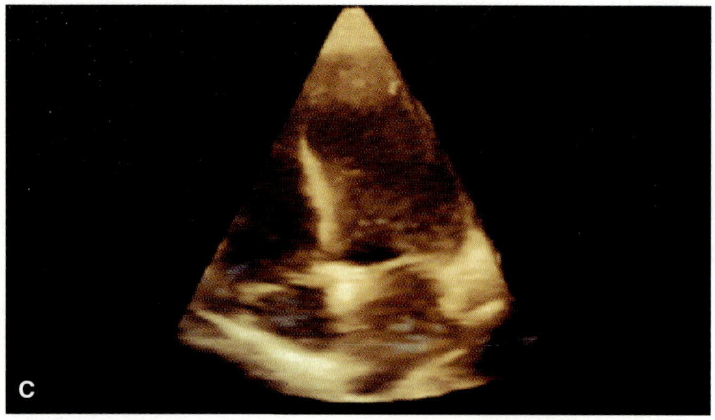

Figure 6C: Mechanical complications of myocardial infarction: Panel on left depicting ventricular septal rupture in the left ventricular apex in a patient with anterior wall myocardial infarction

LV SYSTOLIC ASYNCHRONY

Cardiac resynchronization therapy (CRT) consisting of bi-ventricular pacing has been shown to improve hemodynamics and increase exercise tolerance and quality of life in selected patients with advanced heart failure.[6] Different techniques exist for assessing suitability of patients for resynchronization therapy and for subsequent optimization of pacing parameters. QRS duration (>120 ms) is one of three criteria currently being used to select patients for CRT procedures (the other two criteria are EF < 35% and NYHA class III or IV). QRS-based methods are widely used but fail to take account of all factors influencing mechanical timing and ventricular function and have been shown to select a significant number of patients (up to 30%) who subsequently fail to respond to CRT. Tissue Doppler-based methods such as the TDI Asynchrony Index[34] are promising but are technically demanding, angle and operator dependent, and fail to provide rapid concomitant assessment of global volume and ejection fraction. 3D echo offers an approach which combines accurate determination of delayed contraction sites and mechanical dyssynchrony together with global LV function data. 3D assessment of regional time-volume curves provides additional data for hemodynamic evaluation by allowing measurement of true ventricular regional volumes. Several studies have demonstrated that generation of time volume curves representing LV volume changes over the heart cycle is feasible and accurate and allows calculation of indices such as the SDI (systolic dyssynchrony index) for detailed quantitative analysis of LV performance even in patients with LV dysfunction[34-36] (see Figure 4). Regional timing comparisons based on LV volume curves can now be performed with even greater

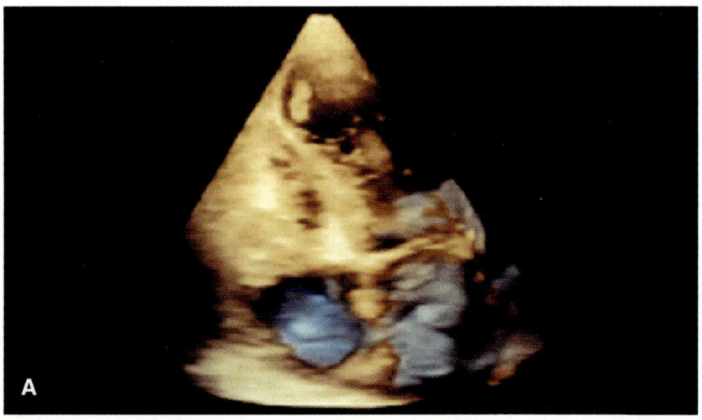

Figure 6A: Showing left ventricular apical thrombus in a patient with LV apical aneurysm who had massive anterior wall myocardial infarction

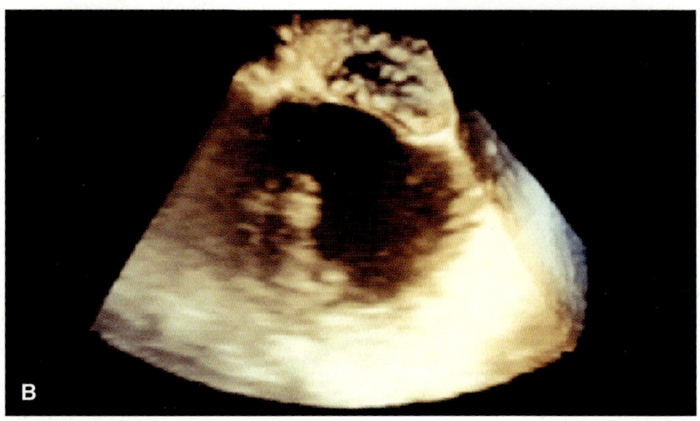

Figure 6B: Transesophageal echocardiogram in a patient with submitral aneurysm and inferior wall myocardial infarction

confidence thanks to temporal resolution enhancements offering Live 3D Echo frame rates up to 80 frames per second.

In patients with LBBB, mechanical dyssynchrony was easy to obtain and to reproduce with RT3DE and the post-processing software. In healthy volunteers, mild mechanical dyssynchrony was observed, in asymptomatic LBBB patients intermediate mechanical dyssynchrony was observed, although not significantly different from healthy volunteers, and in symptomatic LBBB patients, severe mechanical dyssynchrony was observed, which differed significantly from healthy volunteers and asymptomatic LBBB patients.[37]

REFERENCES

1. Weiss JL, Eaton LW, Kallman CH, et al. Accuracy of volume determination by two-dimensional echocardiography: defining requirements under controlled conditions in the ejecting canine left ventricle. Circulation 1983;67:889-95.
2. Raichlen JS, Trivedi SS, Herman GT, et al. Dynamic three-dimensional reconstruction of the left ventricle from two-dimensional echocardiograms. J Am Coll Cardiol 1986;8:364-70.
3. King DL, Harrison MR, King DL Jr, et al. Improved reproducibility of left atrial and left ventricular measurements by guided three-dimensional echocardiography. J Am Coll Cardiol 1992;20:1238-45.
4. Gopal AS, Keller AM, Rigling R, et al. Left ventricular volume and endocardial surface area by three-dimensional echocardiography: comparison with two-dimensional echocardiography and nuclear magnetic resonance imaging in normal subjects. J Am Coll Cardiol 1993;22:258-70.
5. Sapin PM, Schroder KM, Gopal AS, et al. Comparison of two- and three-dimensional echocardiography with cineventriculography for measurement of left ventricular volume in patients. J Am Coll Cardiol 1994;24:1054-63.
6. Hajo Müller, Caroline Frangos, et al. Measurement of left ventricular ejection fraction by real time 3D echocardiography in patients with severe systolic dysfunction: comparison with radionuclide angiography. Echocardiography 2010;27:58-63.
7. Jiang L, Morrissey R, Handschumacher MD, et al. Quantitative three-dimensional reconstruction of left ventricular volume with complete borders detected by acoustic quantification underestimates volume. Am Heart J 1996;131:553-9.
8. Sapin PM, Schroeder KM, Gopal AS, et al. Three-dimensional echocardiography: limitations of apical biplane imaging for measurement of left ventricular volume. J Am Soc Echocardiogr 1995;8:576-84.
9. Gopal AS, Schnellbaecher MJ, Shen Z, et al. Freehand three-dimensional echocardiography for determination of left ventricular volume and mass in patients with abnormal ventricles: comparison with magnetic resonance imaging. J Am Soc Echocardiogr 1997;10:853-61.
10. Gopal AS, Keller AM, Shen Z, et al. Three-dimensional echocardiography:in vitro and in vivo validation of left ventricular mass and comparison with conventional echocardiographic methods. J Am Coll Cardiol 1994;24:504-13.
11. Sapin PM, Gopal AS, Clarke GB, et al. Three-dimensional echocardiography compared to two-dimensional echocardiography for measurement of left ventricular mass anatomic validation in an open chest canine model. Am J Hypertens 1996;9:467-74.
12. Altmann K, Shen Z, Boxt LM, et al. Comparison of three dimensional echocardiographic assessment of volume, mass, and function in children with functionally single left ventricles with two-dimensional echocardiography and magnetic resonance imaging. Am J Cardiol 1997;80:1060-5.
13. Levine RA, Handschumacher MD, Sanfilippo AJ, et al. Three-dimensional echocardiographic reconstruction of the mitral valve, with implications for the diagnosis of mitral valve prolapse. Circulation 1989;80:589-98.
14. Roberto M Lang, Victor Mor-Avi, Lissa Sugeng, et al. Three-dimensional echocardiography: the benefits of the additional dimensions. J Am Coll Cardiol 2006;48:2053-69.
15. Victor Mor-Avi, Roberto M Lang. Three-Dimensional echocardiographic evaluation of the heart chambers: size, function, and mass. Cardiol Clin 2007;25:241-51.
16. Jacobs LD, Salgo IS, Goonewardena S, et al. Rapid online quantification of left ventricular volume from real-time three-dimensional echocardiographic data. Eur Heart J 2006;27:460-8.
17. Arai K, Hozumi T, Matsumura Y, et al. Accuracy of measurement of left ventricular volume and ejection fraction by new real-time three-dimensional echocardiography in patients with wall motion abnormalities secondary to myocardial infarction. Am J Cardiol 2004;94:552-8.
18. Jenkins C, Bricknell K, HanekomL, et al. Reproducibility and accuracy of echocardiographic measurements of left ventricular parameters using real-time three-dimensional echocardiography. J Am Coll Cardiol 2004;44:878-86.

19. Keller AM, Gopal AS, King DL. Left and right atrial volume by freehand three-dimensional echocardiography: in vivo validation using magnetic resonance imaging. Eur J Echocardiogr 2000;1:55-65.
20. Kawai J, Tanabe K, Wang CL, et al. Comparison of left atrial size by freehand scanning three-dimensional echocardiography and two dimensional echocardiography. Eur J Echocardiogr 2004;5:18-24.
21. Jiang L, Handschumacher MD, Hibberd MG, et al. Three dimensional echocardiographic reconstruction of right ventricular volume: in vitro comparison with two-dimensional methods. J Am Soc Echocardiogr 1994;7:150-8.
22. Dorosz JL, Bolson EL, Waiss MS, et al. Three-dimensional visual guidance improves the accuracy of calculating right ventricular volume with two-dimensional echocardiography. J Am Soc Echocardiogr 2003;16:675-81.
23. Kjaergaard J, Petersen CL, Kjaer A, et al. Evaluation of right ventricular volume and function by 2D and 3D echocardiography compared to MRI. Eur J Echocardiogr 2005.
24. Corsi C, Lang RM, Veronesi F, et al. Volumetric quantification of global and regional left ventricular function from real-time three-dimensional echocardiographic images. Circulation 2005;112:1161-70.
25. Takeuchi M, Otani S, Weinert L, et al. Comparison of contrast-enhanced real-time live 3-dimensional dobutamine stress echocardiography with contrast 2-dimensional echo-cardiography for detecting stress-induced wall-motion abnormalities. J Am Soc Echocardiogr 2006;19:294-9.
26. Luigi P Badano, Denisa Muraru, Fausto Rigo, et al. High volume-rate three-dimensional stress echocardiography to assess inducible myocardial ischemia: a feasibility study. J Am Soc Echocardiogr 2010;23:628-35.
27. Buck T, Plicht B, Hunold P, et al. Broad-beam spectral Doppler sonification of the vena contracta using matrix array technology: a new solution for semiautomated quantification of mitral regurgitant flow volume and orifice area. J Am Coll Cardiol. 2005 Mar 1;45(5):770-9.
28. Sugeng L, Weinert L, Lammertin G, et al. Accuracy of volumetric mitral valve orifice area measurements using a transthoracic rapid free-hand scanning method: comparison with conventional non-invasive and invasive methods. J Am Society of Echocardiography 2003;16:1292-1300.
29. Zamorano J, Sugeng L, Cordeiro P, et al. Real-time 3D echocardiography for rheumatic mitral valve stenosis evaluation: an accurate and novel approach. J Am Coll Cardiol 2004;42(11):2091-6.
30. Otsuji Y, Handschumacher MD, Schwammenthal E, et al. Insights from three-dimensional echocardiography into the mechanism of functional mitral regurgitation: direct in vivo demonstration of altered leaflet tethering geometry. Circulation 1997;96:1999e2008.
31. Caiani EG, Coon P, Corsi C, et al. Dual triggering improves the accuracy of left ventricular volume measurements by contrast-enhanced real-time 3-dimensional echocardiography. J Am Soc Echocardiogr 2005;18:1292-8.
32. Corsi C, Coon P, Goonewardena S, et al. Quantification of regional left ventricular function from real-time 3D echocardiography in patients with poor acoustic windows: effects of contrast enhancement tested against cardiac magnetic resonance. J Am Soc Echocardiogr 2006;19:886-93.
33. Mor-Avi V, Caiani EG, Collins KA, et al. Combined assessment of myocardial perfusion and regional left ventricular function by analysis of contrast-enhanced power modulation images. Circulation 2001;104:352-7.
34. Zhang Q, Yu CM, Fung J, et al. Assessment of the effect of cardiac resynchronization therapy on intraventricular mechanical synchronicity by regional volumetric changes. Am J Cardiol 2005;95:126-8.
35. Joseph A. Horstman, MDa, Mark J Monaghan. Intraventricular Dyssynchrony Assessment by Real-Time Three-Dimensional Echocardiography. Cardiol Clin 25 (2007) 253-60.
36. Wei Cui, Katheryn Gambetta, Frank Zimmerman, et al. Real-time three-dimensional echocardiographic assessment of left ventricular systolic dyssynchrony in healthy children. J Am Soc Echocardiogr 2010;23:1153-9
37. Jeroen van Dijk, Pieter A Dijkmans, Marco JW Gotte, et al. Evaluation of global left ventricular function and mechanical dyssynchrony in patients with an asymptomatic left bundle branch block: a real-time 3D echocardiography study. European Journal of Echocardiography 2008;9:40-6.

CHAPTER 7

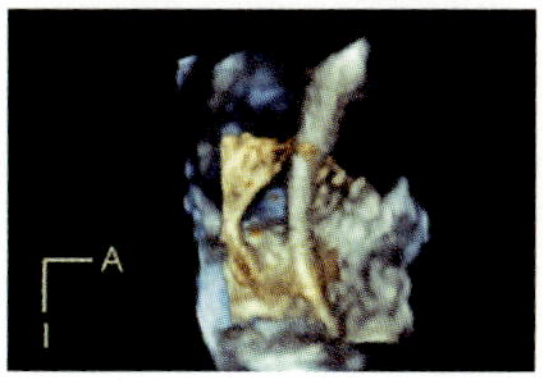

Three-Dimensional Echocardiography in Congenital Heart Defects

Girish S Shirali, Raman Krishna Kumar

INTRODUCTION

Complex intracardiac anatomy and spatial relationships are inherent to congenital heart defects (CHD). Beginning over thirty years ago and until recently, the clinician's ability to image the heart by echocardiography has been limited to two-dimensional techniques.[1] In the interim, there have been important advances in two-dimensional echocardiography (2DE). Improving transducer technology, beam-forming and miniaturization have led to significant improvements in spatial and temporal resolution using 2DE. However, 2DE has fundamental limitations. The very nature of a 2DE slice, which has no thickness, necessitates the use of multiple orthogonal 'sweeps'. The echocardiographer then mentally reconstructs the anatomy, and uses the structure of the report to express this mentally reconstructed vision. This means that the only three-dimensional image of the heart is the 'virtual image' that exists in the echocardiographer's mind, and is then translated into words. It is not easy for an untrained—albeit interested—observer to understand the images obtained in the course of a sweep: expert interpretation is required. Since myocardial motion occurs in three dimensions, 2DE techniques inherently do not lend themselves to accurate quantitation.

Recognition of these limitations of 2DE led to burgeoning research and clinical interest in the modality of 3DE. Early reconstructive approaches were based on 2DE image acquisitions that were subsequently stacked and aligned based on phases of the cardiac cycle, in order to recreate a 3DE dataset.[2-5] While these approaches proved to be accurate, the need for time and offline processing equipment imposed fundamental limitations on their clinical applicability. In 1990, von Ramm and Smith published their early results with a matrix array transducer that provided real-time images of the heart in three dimensions.[6] While this was an important breakthrough, this transducer was unable to be steered in the third (elevation) dimension. Over the past five years, dramatic technological advances have facilitated the ability to perform live 3DE scanning, including the ability to steer the beam in three dimensions and to render the image in real time.[7]

3DE TECHNOLOGY

Technologic advances that have facilitated the maturation of 3DE techniques include the following:

Matrix transducers Beam forming and steering in three spatial dimensions

Display of three-dimensional information Software for quantification

MATRIX TRANSDUCERS

Two important advances in transducer technology, namely the organization of elements and the use of novel piezoelectric materials, have been the structural basis for improvements in 3DE matrix transducers.

ELEMENTS

Contemporary matrix-array transducers comprise as many elements in the elevational dimension as they do in the azimuthal dimension, with over 60 elements in each of these dimensions. While the elements are arranged in a two-dimensional grid, this array generates 3DE images. In order to be able to steer in the elevational plane, each element must be electrically independent from all other elements, and each element must be electrically active. The technology and electrical circuitry to electrically insulate and connect each element became commercially available in 2002. As a result, the contemporary matrix array transducer consists of thousands of electrically active elements that independently steer a scan line left and right, as well as up and down.

PIEZOELECTRIC MATERIALS

The piezoelectric material in an ultrasound transducer is a fundamental determinant of system image quality. Piezoelectric transducer elements are responsible for delivery of ultrasound energy into the scanned tissue and for converting returning ultrasound echoes into electric signals. Their coupling efficiency in converting electrical energy to mechanical energy or vice versa is a key determinant of image quality, Doppler sensitivity and penetration. To create an overall piezoelectric effect, these elements must be subject to the application of an external electric field to align dipoles within polycrystalline materials. For almost forty years, a ceramic polycrystalline material, PZT (lead-zirconate-titanate) or PZT composites, has been the standard piezoelectric material used in medical imaging. This material is a uniform powder that is mixed with an organic binder; the resulting compound is baked into a dense polycrystalline structure. At its best, it achieves ~ 70% alignment of dipoles due to imperfect alignment of the individual dipoles. This leads to a corresponding constraint in the electromechanical coupling efficiency of the material.

One example of new piezoelectric material involves growing crystals from a molten ceramic material, resulting in a homogenous crystal with fewer defects, lower losses and no grain boundaries.[8-10] When these crystals are poled at the preferred orientation(s), near perfect alignment of dipoles (~100%) is achievable resulting in dramatically enhanced electromechanical properties (Figure 1). The efficiency of conversion of electrical to mechanical energy improves by as much as 68-85% when compared to PZT ceramics currently used in ultrasound transducers. The new piezoelectric materials provide increased bandwidth and sensitivity, resulting in both penetration and high-resolution.

The improved arrangement of atoms in these new piezoelectric materials, and their superior strain energy density, translate into advances in transducer miniaturization. The recent implementation of these advances has led to the availability of a high frequency matrix 3DE transthoracic transducer that has dramatically enhanced the applicability of 3DE to pediatric populations.[11,12]

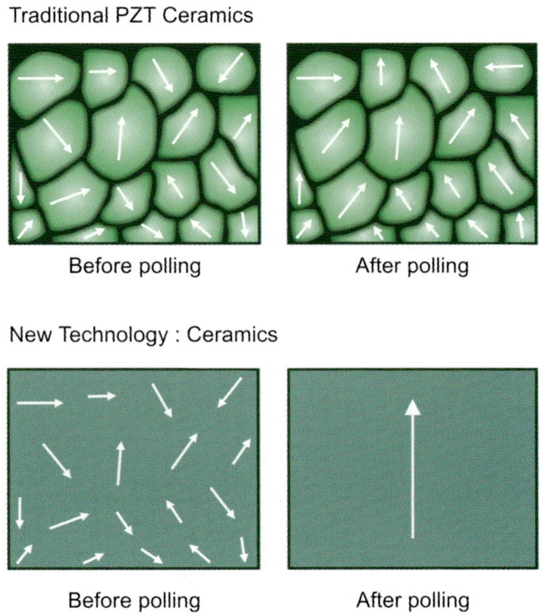

Figure 1: The top panel shows imperfect alignment of dipoles in traditional piezoelectric (PZT) crystals after poling (application of an external electrical field). The bottom panel shows almost perfect alignment of dipoles in new piezoelectric material

THREE-DIMENSIONAL BEAM FORMING AND STEERING

Beam forming constitutes the steering and focusing of transmitted and received scan lines. For 3DE, this means that beam former must be steered both in the azimuthal and elevational planes. This is achieved both in the ultrasound system and within the transducer itself, using highly specialized integrated circuits to create a 3D trapezoid of acoustic information that is processed. These 3DE data are summed, processed and finally placed into rectangular space using a 3D scan converter.

DISPLAY OF 3DE

Two-dimensional computer displays consist of rows and blocks of picture elements, termed pixels, that comprise a 2D image. In contrast, a 3DE data set consists of bricks of pixels, termed volume elements or voxels. However, even for a 3DE data set, the two-dimensional nature of the display imposes restrictions on the ability to appreciate depth. As shown initially by the ancient Greeks and subsequently rediscovered during the renaissance, perspective is used to simulate the appearance of 3D depth, providing objects the appearance of being close to or deeper/further away from the screen. The process of adding perspective is done by casting a light beam through the collection of voxels. The light beam either hits enough tissue so as to render it opaque, or it keeps shining through transparent voxels so as to render it transparent. More recent algorithms apply different hues to the front of the data set (nearest to the screen) as opposed to voxels that are far from the screen (Figure 2). The user has the ability to rotate and tilt the data set on the computer screen. Tools are available to 'cut away' interfering structures, thus performing 'virtual dissection'.

SOFTWARE FOR QUANTIFICATION

Quantification requires segmentation of structures of interest from the acquired data. Since myocardial motion occurs in three spatial dimensions, 2DE planes are inherently incapable of capturing the entire motion.

Two-dimensional techniques for quantitation are based on geometric formulas that rely on assumptions regarding the shapes of cardiac structures. However, these assumptions are frequently incorrect. In contrast, 3DE acquisitions include the entire extent of the structure, thus minimizing the possibility of foreshortening of the apex or any geometric assumptions regarding shape.

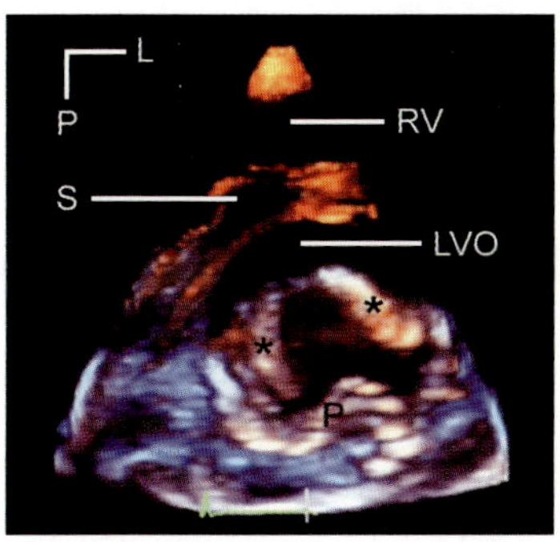

Figure 2: This is a parasternal short axis image of a cleft in the anterior mitral leaflet. Asterisks mark the edges of the cleft. A tissue colorization map has been applied to the image. This has the effect of coloring tissues in the near field (near to either the transducer or the front of the 3D image) orange. Tissues in the far filed are colored blue. This is a dynamic after-effect, which means that as the operator rotates, tilts or otherwise manipulates the image, the color effect correspondingly changes in real-time. L, left; LVO, left ventricular outflow tract; P, posterior; RV, right ventricle; S, septum

Three-dimensional quantitative software tools have the potential to quantify cardiac structures accurately regardless of their shape. Advances in the software tools for processing 3DE datasets have mirrored the rapid advances in transducer technology that have occurred over the past five years.

3DE volumetric techniques rely on definition of chamber cavities, that is, the blood-endocardium interface. The software constructs this interface by using a process known as surface rendering, and represents it as a mesh of points and lines. This software-generated mesh is calculated for every frame of acquisition, thus providing a moving cast of the cavity of the ventricle during the cardiac cycle. Since this is digital data, it provides for ease of computation of global and regional volumes, synchrony as well as parametric displays of endocardial excursion and timing of contraction (Figure 3).

3DE quantification tools for the left ventricle (LV) are more technologically advanced than for other cardiac structures. Until recently, 3DE LV quantification tools employed the method of disk summation. With improvements in computing speeds and programming, newer tools have been developed to provide instantaneous tracking of the blood pool—endocardium interface at each frame of acquisition. This provides a surface-rendered model that is displayed as a mesh of lines and points. However, these approaches are still based on some basic 3D geometric assumptions regarding left ventricular shape, and therefore their application cannot be extended to the right ventricle or to univentricular hearts. Given the complex shape and architecture of the right ventricle, it is not surprising that tools for quantifying right ventricular (RV) volume have been slower to mature. Until very recently, these tools utilized the method of disks for volumetrics.[13] Novel software now provides instantaneous tracking of the blood pool—endocardium interface at each frame of acquisition (Figure 4).

This yields a surface-rendered model that is displayed as a mesh of lines and points.[14]

Quantitative software for the mitral valve provides the ability to perform sophisticated analyses of the nonplanar shape of the mitral annulus and to measure 3D structures including annular diameters, commissural lengths, leaflet

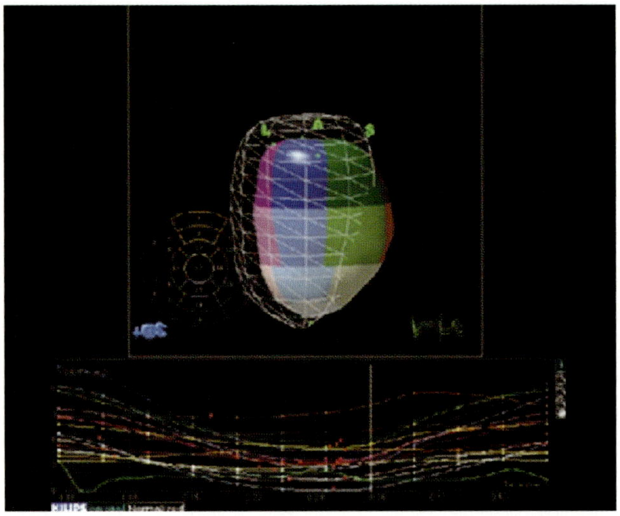

Figure 3: Software for processing 3DE enables quantitation of left ventricular volumes throughout the cardiac cycle, providing end-diastolic and end-systolic volume as well as ejection fraction. The mesh represents left ventricular volume at end-diastole. The cast of the left ventricular cavity consists of segments of varying colors, each of which represents a sub-volume of the ventricular cavity based on the American Society of Echocardiography 16-segment model. The change in volume of each sub-volume is represented graphically, with time on the X axis and volume on the Y axis

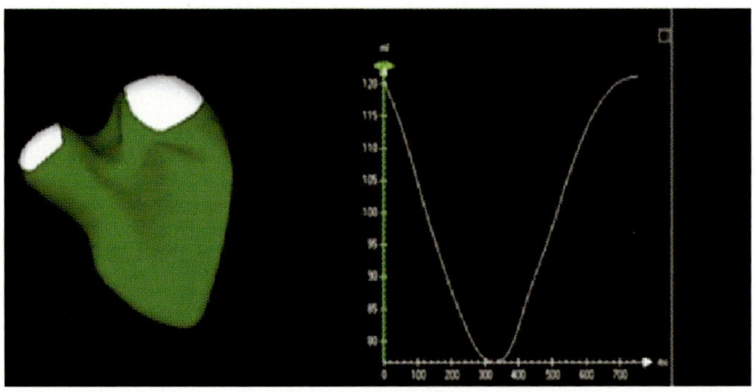

Figure 4: Novel software provides the ability to measure right ventricular volume throughout the cardiac cycle. This yields a surface-rendered model that is displayed as a mesh of lines and points. The change in volume is represented graphically, with time on the X axis and volume on the Y axis

surface areas.[15,16] Quantitative techniques have also been developed to provide volumetric measurements of 3D color flow using non-aliased color flow data.

MODES OF 3DE

Electronically-steered 3DE systems have two major modes of scanning: live and EKG-gated. The live mode is the only one where the system scans in 3D real-time. A defining characteristic of this mode is: if the transducer comes off the chest, the image disappears. The live 3D mode can also be operated within a three-dimensionally shaped zoom box. Live 3DE modes provide narrow (20 to 30 degrees in the elevation plane) datasets that have high voxel density. Live 3DE can be obtained on patients with arrhythmias or with an active precordium with no potential for motion or stitch artifacts.

EKG-gated modes are required to provide wider volumes while maintaining adequate frame rates (Figure 5).

Gating allows for anywhere from four to eight smaller volumes to be stitched together to generate volumes that are greater than 90 degrees wide in the elevation plane, at frame rates exceeding 30 Hz. Gated modes have comparatively lower voxel density, and are subject to both motion and stitch artifacts. Recent enhancements have improved the ability to acquire gated full volume data among patients with arrhythmias. Gated modes are available using grayscale or with color flow Doppler.

Contemporary 3DE systems provide the user with tools to vary frame rate, 3D volume size and image resolution. Increasing the requirement in one of these causes a drop in the other two, all things being equal.

Given the potential for motion and stitch artifacts with gated modes and the need for high spatial and temporal resolution, it has been our practice to use live 3DE to delineate anatomy. We reserve the use of gated modes for the following:

Complicated cardiac anatomy that requires extensive offline cropping Targets that do not fit within a live 3DE window Quantitation of chamber volumes 3DE color flow demonstrations of regurgitant jets or shunt flows.

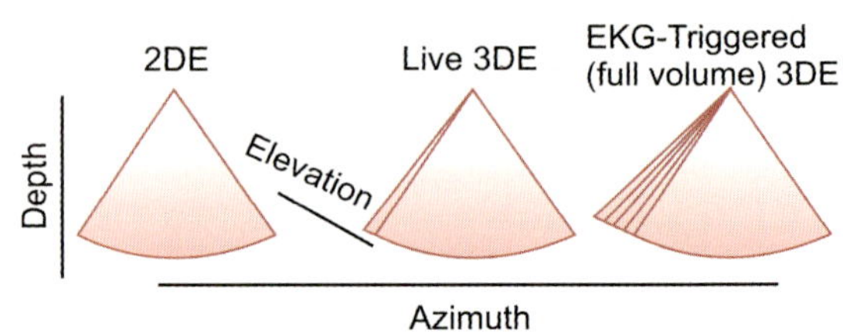

Figure 5: Depicts the differences between 2D, live 3D and full-volume (EKG-triggered) 3DE. Conventional 2DE is shown in the left panel. Live 3DE imaging (center panel) adds the elevation plane. The shape of the image is therefore trapezoidal rather than pie-shaped. The right panel depicts EKG-triggered (full volume) 3DE imaging, which provides a wider trapezoid

MODES

Live 3DE imaging has been commercially available for transthoracic and fetal applications since 2002. Live 3DE transesophageal echocardiographic imaging became commercially available in 2007. This has yielded images never before seen on the beating heart (Figure 6). We anticipate that continuing improvements in transducer technology and the wider applicability of advances in piezoelectrics will enable the application of 3DE technology to an ever-increasing range of patient sizes, windows and applications.

CLINICAL APPLICATIONS IN CONGENITAL HEART DISEASE

3DE imaging has three broad areas of clinical application among patients with congenital heart disease: visualization of morphology, volumetric quantitation of chamber sizes and flows, and image-guided interventions.

VISUALIZATION OF MORPHOLOGY

Dating from an early stage in the development of 3DE technology, the structural complexity that is inherent to congenital heart disease has been identified as fertile substrate for exploration using 3DE.[17-19]

THE ATRIOVENTRICULAR VALVES

3DE is valuable in delineating the morphology of the atrioventricular valves. Espinola-Zavaleta et al, described the role of 3DE in delineating congenital abnormalities of the mitral valve.[20] Lu et al, demonstrated that 3DE allowed comprehensive assessment of the anatomy of double orifice mitral valve.[21] Rawlins et al, demonstrated the additive value of 3DE and improved image quality using intraoperative epicardial 3DE to delineate the anatomy of atrioventricular (AV) valves.[22] Seliem et al, studied 41 patients with AV valve abnormalities and found that 3DE imaging was helpful in delineating the morphology of the valve leaflets and their chordal attachments, the subchordal apparatus, the mechanism and origin of regurgitation, and the geometry of the regurgitant volume.[23] Vettųkatil et al, examined the role of 3DE in patients with Ebstein's anomaly of the tricuspid valve. They demonstrated that 3DE provided clear visualization of the morphology of the valve leaflets, including the extent of their formation, the level of their attachment, and their degree of coaptation. They were also able to visualize the mechanism of regurgitation or stenosis.[24]

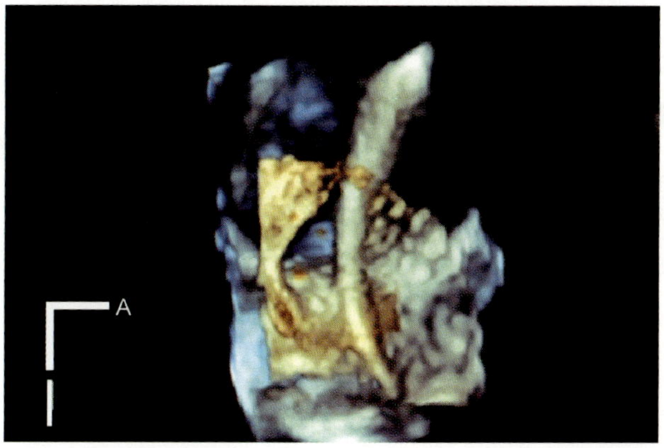

Figure 6: Live 3D transesophageal echocardiography demonstrates a catheter passing through a large atrial septal defect. The viewing perspective is unique: the observer is virtually located within the left atrium, looking rightwards. A, anterior; I, inferior

ATRIOVENTRICULAR SEPTAL DEFECT

Hlavacek et al, studied 52 datasets on 51 patients with atrioventricular septal defects (AVSD) and showed that gated 3DE views could be cropped to obtain en face views of the atrial and ventricular septa.[25] These views provide a clear understanding of the relationships of the bridging leaflets to the septal structures (Figures 7 and 8). These views have been useful to determine the precise location of the interventricular communication relative to the bridging leaflets, and to demonstrate how these relationships determine the level of shunting (atrial, ventricular or both atrial and ventricular). They found that 3DE on unrepaired balanced AVSD and repaired AVSD with residual lesions was more often additive/useful (33/36; 92%) than on repaired AVSD without residual lesions or unbalanced AVSD (9/16 (56%), P = 0.009). 3DE was additive or useful in all 3 patients with unbalanced AVSD being considered for biventricular repair. Useful information obtained by 3DE included: precise characterization of mitral regurgitation and leaflet anatomy, substrate for subaortic stenosis, valve anatomy, and presence and location of additional septal defects.

THE ATRIAL AND VENTRICULAR SEPTA

Tantengco et al, showed that 3DE reconstructions provided unique en face views of atrial and ventricular septal defects.[26] Cheng et al, studied 38 patients with atrial and/or ventricular septal defects using 3DE, and compared their results to 2DE and surgical findings. They demonstrated novel 3DE views of both atrial and ventricular septal defects and improved accuracy of quantification of the size of the defect by 3DE compared to 2DE (r = 0.92 vs. r = 0.69).[27] This approach has also been used to demonstrate the morphology of muscular ventricular septal defects.[28] We have found live 3DE to be of great value in evaluating complex malformations of the outflow tract that involve malalignment of the outlet septum.

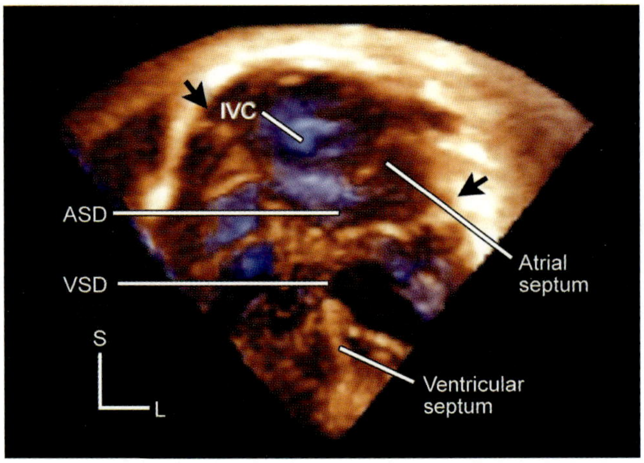

Figure 7: This is an apical four chamber 3D echocardiogram in a patient with atrioventricular septal defect. Arrowheads mark the hinges of the common atrioventricular junction. The bridging leaflets divide the defect into an interatrial (ASD) and interventricular (VSD) component. Note the posterior location of the inferior vena cava orifice (IVCJ relative to the septal structures. L, left; S, superior

THE AORTIC ARCH, PULMONARY ARTERIES AND AORTOPULMONARY SHUNTS

3DE color flow Doppler has been used to provide echocardiographic 'angiograms' of flow patterns in the aortic arch (coarctation of the aorta), the branch pulmonary arteries (the Lecompte maneuver) and across Blalock-Taussig shunts.[29] These authors examined echocardiographic 'angiograms' in 26 patients (Figure 9). 3DE provided additional diagnostic information in 10 of 26 patients (38%). In 17 of 26 patients (65%), validation of the 3DE diagnosis was available at surgery, cardiac catheterization, MRI or CT angiography.

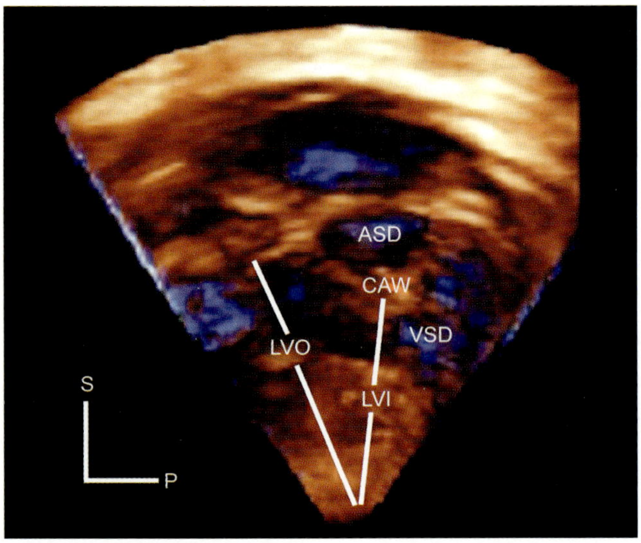

Figure 8: This is an en face view of the left ventricular aspect of the ventricular septum in a patient with atrioventricular septal defect. The free walls of the left atrium and left ventricle have been cropped. The viewer is looking from left to right. This view demonstrates the left ventricular inflow-outflow disproportion that characterizes AV septal defect. Note the crescentic inferior margin of the atrial septum, and the scooped-out edge of the interventricular septum. This view provides excellent anatomic detail regarding the relationships between the bridging leaflets of the common AV valve (CAW) and the septal structures. P, posterior; S, superior

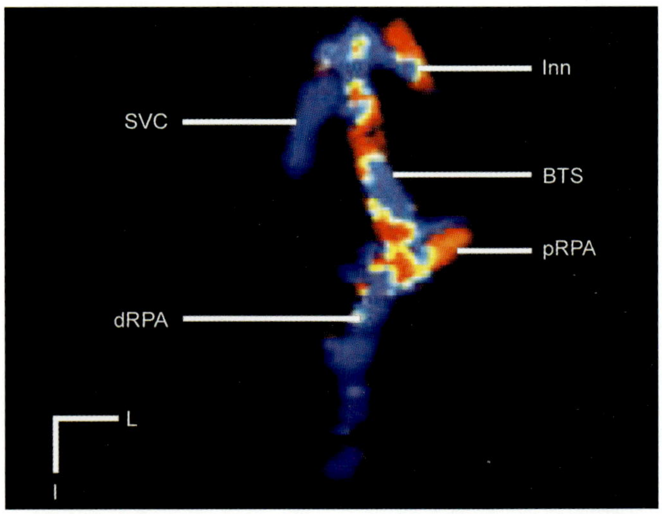

Figure 9: This is a 3DE color flow, ECG-triggered (full volume) acquisition demonstrating a right sided Blalock-Taussig shunt (BTS). The grayscale image has been suppressed, thus providing an echocardiographic angiogram. The shunt is seen in its entirety from its origin from the innominate artery (Inn) to its insertion. The proximal and distal right pulmonary artery (pRPA and dRPA respectively) are well seen. Note the proximity of the superior vena cava (SVC) to the cranial end of the shunt. This dataset can be rotated, tilted and examined in an infinite number of planes in order to delineate the location of stenosis. I, inferior; L, left

THE AORTIC VALVE AND OUTFLOW TRACT

Sadagopan et al, examined the role of 3DE in 8 children who subsequently underwent surgery for congenital aortic valvar stenosis. They showed that 3DE was accurate in providing measurements of aortic valve annulus, number of valve leaflets, in identifying sites of fusion of the leaflets as well as nodules and excrescences that characterized dysplastic valves.[30] Bharucha et al, studied 16 patients with subaortic stenosis. Using a form of 3DE reconstruction known as multiplanar reconstruction, which provides access to an unlimited number of 2DE planes, they demonstrated abnormalities of mitral valve leaflet or chordal apparatus attachments (14 patients), abnormal ventricular muscle band (11 patients) and abnormal increased aorto-mitral separation (2 patients).[31]

CHARACTERIZATION OF LEFT VENTRICULAR NONCOMPACTION

Baker et al, evaluated 4 patients with left ventricular non-compaction using 3DE.[32] They found that 3DE enabled diagnosis and provided detailed characterization of the affected myocardium, including easy visualization of entire trabecular projections, intertrabecular recesses, endocardial borders and wall motion abnormalities of the affected myocardium. 3DE enabled easy differentiation between compacted and noncompacted portions of the myocardium.

QUANTITATION OF CHAMBER DIMENSIONS, VALVE APPARATUS, FUNCTION AND FLOWS

LEFT VENTRICULAR VOLUMETRICS

3DE quantitation provides both proven and potential value for pediatric echocardiography. Bu et al compared 3DE measurements of LV volumetrics to those obtained using MRI.[33] Their study showed that 3DE measurements of LV end-systolic volume, end-diastolic volume, mass, stroke volume and ejection fraction in children using a rapid full volume acquisition strategy are feasible, reproducible and comparable with MRI measurements. They found good correlations between the two methods, but a tendency towards mild underestimation of volumes by 3DE. Interestingly, estimates of ejection fraction were in closer agreement. Baker et al evaluated the feasibility of 3DE LV volumetrics, as well as the resource utilization, learning curve, inter- and intra-observer reproducibility of this technique. The study design involved 15 datasets and four observers who had varying degrees of (self-rated) experience with 3DE quantitation.[34] They found that in 59 of 60 instances, observers were able to obtain 3D LV ejection fraction in less than 3 minutes (median time 1 minute and 27 seconds). They demonstrated a learning curve for the observer with the lowest level of self-rated experience. Their study also showed excellent inter- and intra-observer reproducibility for 3DE LV volumetrics.

LEFT VENTRICULAR MASS

Studies in adults have validated 3DE as an accurate method for measuring LV mass.[35-37] While studies in children have been limited in number and scope, Riehle et al recently demonstrated excellent correlations between LV mass measured by 3DE and MRI.[38]

LEFT VENTRICULAR DYSSYNCHRONY

The 3DE approach to measuring intra-LV dyssynchrony utilizes the American Society of Echocardiography's 16-segment model of the LV.[39] It measures the time of each subvolume from maximal (end-diastolic) volume to minimal volume, and the standard deviation of these time intervals. The higher is the value of the standard deviation, the higher the implied degree of intra-LV dyssynchrony. Baker et al, examined the association between LV dysfunction and intra-LV dyssynchrony in children using 3DE.[40] They studied 9 children with dilated cardiomyopathy and an equal number of age- and body size-matched normals. They found that normal patients had 3DE dyssynchrony indices that were below 3%. Among children with dilated cardiomyopathy, there was a clear threshold value of LV ejection fraction (EF): at an LVEF below 35–40%, intra-LV dyssynchrony was the rule. In contrast, patients whose LVEF was higher than 40% exhibited no significant dyssynchrony.

RIGHT VENTRICULAR VOLUMETRICS

Until recently, the accuracy of 3DE measurement of RV volume and ejection fraction had not been evaluated. This is unsurprising given the complex architecture of the right ventricle, and the technical difficulty of imaging it adequately. Recently, Gopal et al reported a large series of adults who underwent RV volumetric measurements using MRI and 3DE using the disk summation method.[13] Niemann et al studied RV volumes by 3DE using a new and robust protocol that utilizes multiplanar reconstruction and tracing with semi-automated border detection in 16 children with congenital heart disease.[14] They found excellent correlations between MRI and 3DE for measurement of RV volumes and ejection fraction. As these tools become more widely available, user-friendly and accurate, we may well see the emergence of a new paradigm in the use of echocardiographic parameters as surrogate outcome measures in clinical trials of medications and pacing strategies. The Pediatric Heart Disease Clinical Research Network is examining RV volumetrics as a secondary outcome measure in the single ventricle reconstruction study, which examines for differences between initial shunt type on survival following the Norwood procedure for neonates with hypoplastic left heart syndrome (unpublished,http://www.pediatricheartnetwork.org/svrforhealth careproviders.asp).

VISUALIZATION AND QUANTITATION OF 3DE COLOR FLOW

Multiplanar reconstruction tools provide the ability to not only visualize but also to trace and measure the area of valvar regurgitant orifices at the level of the vena contracta. While this technique is new and has not been validated, it has been shown to be feasible, and has already yielded new insights into the shape of regurgitant jets, and holds promise as a tool to enhance the echocardiographer's ability to serially quantify valve regurgitation.[41-43] Pemberton et al, developed a technique for quantifying non-aliased 3DE color flow jets *in vitro*.[44] They validated this technique on open-chested pigs; when compared to measurements obtained from flow probes positioned on the ascending aorta, they obtained excellent correlations between the two methods.[45] They compared 143 individual measurements of cardiac output and found excellent correlation between the two techniques (r2 = 0.93). 3DE quantification of color flow has recently been validated in adults by comparison to cardiac outputs obtained by thermodilution.[46] Application of this technique to pathologic states could lead to potentially more accurate measurements of regurgitant volumes and fractions.[47]

IMAGE-GUIDED INTERVENTIONS

The high temporal and spatial resolution of trans-thoracic and particularly trans-esophageal echocardiography has ignited interest in the potential uses of live 3DE to guide interventions. Scheurer et al, demonstrated the use of live 3DE to guide the performance of endomyocardial biopsy in children.[48] In their experience, the use of live 3DE guidance was associated with no complications, including no new tricuspid valve leaflet flail or pericardial effusion. 3DE proved to be a reliable noninvasive modality to accurately direct the bioptome to the desired site of biopsy within the right ventricle. As familiarity with this technique increased, the need for fluoroscopic guidance of bioptome manipulation in the right ventricle was minimized. Del Nido et al have extended the concept of image-guided intervention to the very novel approach of epicardial live 3DE-guided, open-chest, closed-heart, off-bypass cardiac surgery.[49-52] They began with *in vitro* validation of the ability of live 3DE to guide the performance of common surgical tasks. More recently, they have undertaken closure of small atrial septal defects in the porcine model using live 3DE guidance. With the recent introduction of live 3D TEE, we have been able to obtain spectacular images of cardiac chambers, septal structures and valves. Live 3D TEE is being used to guide catheter manipulations, trans-septal procedures and closure of atrial septal defects (Figure 10 and 11).[53]

LEARNING CURVE

The learning curve with 3DE is steep but negotiable. Our experience would suggest that the success of 3DE in a program requires advocacy and an investment of time by both echocardiographers and sonographers. The acceptance of 3DE is improving on a global level, albeit at an early stage of the technology cycle. We have developed and implemented an interactive teaching course that utilizes simulations using 3DE datasets with rehearsal and direct mentoring; this has been shown to be useful in overcoming the steep part of the learning curve.[54]

LIMITATIONS

Many of the limitations of 2DE imaging extend to 3D echocardiography. Patients who have poor windows for 2DE examinations are unlikely to have good 3DE windows. Structures that are difficult to visualize by 2DE because they are thin and parallel to the imaging plane, such as the atrial septum in a teenager as viewed from an apical view, will probably remain difficult to visualize from that imaging window by 3DE.

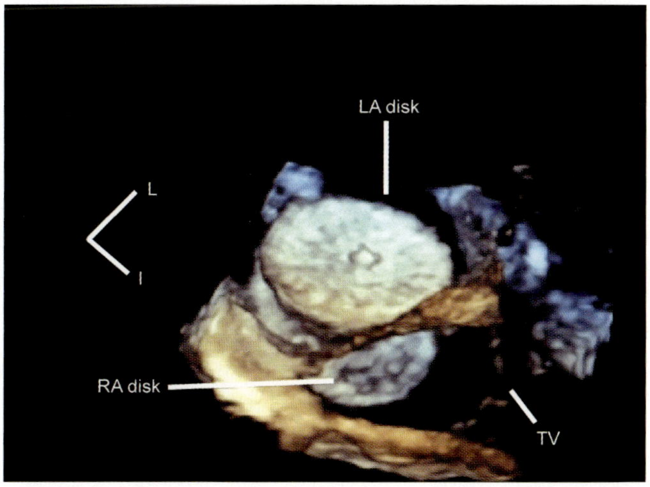

Figure 10: This is a live 3D transesophageal echocardiogram immediately following device closure of a fenestrated atrial septum with a cribriformAmp latzer septal occluder. The viewer is virtually placed inside the left atrium, looking rightwards and posteriorly. The entire left atrial disk of the device is seen, with its central umbilication and the meshwork of metal that constitutes its frame. Part of the inferior portion of the right atrial disk (RAdisk) and the tricuspid valve apparatus (TV) are also seen. I, inferior; L, left

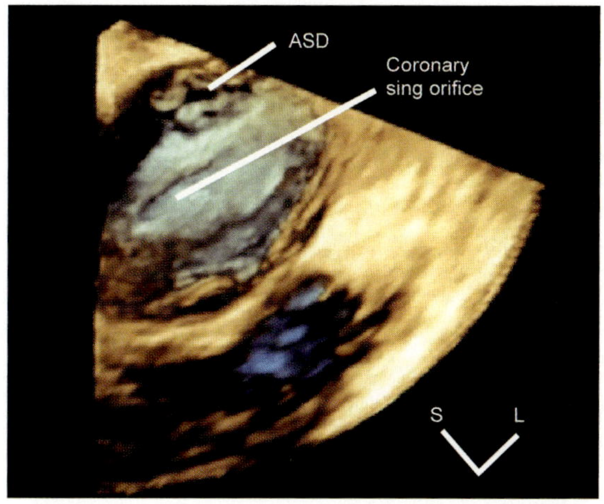

Figure 11: This is a live 3DE transesophageal echocardiogram in a patient with a low secundum atrial septal defect. 2DE imaging demonstrated that the defect was in proximity to the coronary sinus, raising doubts about candidacy for device closure. In this 3DE image, the free walls and appendage of the right atrium have been removed. The viewer is looking posteriorly and leftwards. Note the high resolution of anatomic detail. The atrial septal defect is separated from the coronary sinus orifice by a reasonable distance. Based on the shape and size of the defect, this was felt by 3DE to be a reasonable candidate for device closure, which was successfully accomplished. L, left; S, superior

Given the early stage of development of this technology at the current time, it is unsurprising that governing bodies such as the American Society of Echocardiography have not yet developed formal protocols.

FUTURE DIRECTIONS

Over the next decade, advances in the 3DE arena will involve technical enhancements such as improved image resolution, holographic displays, a wide range of validated software tools for quantification, and enhancements to work flow. New, multi-modality applications will increasingly bring 3DE into the mainstream. Refinements in transducer technology will make high-resolution 3DE available across the spectrum of patient sizes. We anticipate a 3DE TEE probe miniaturized for pediatric usage. With the growing interest in multi-modality imaging, 3DE volumetric data will eventually be integrated with the pressure data that is available during cardiac catheterization, yielding pressure-volume loops that can be obtained as a matter of routine clinical practice.

REFERENCES

1. Tajik AJ, Seward JB, Hagler DJ, et al. Two-dimensional real-time ultrasonic imaging of the heart and great vessels: Technique, image orientation, structure identification and validation. Mayo Clin Proc 1978;53:271-303.
2. Ariet M, Geiser EA, Lupkiewicz SM, et al. Evaluation of a three-dimensional reconstruction to compute left ventricular volume and mass. Am J Cardiol 1984;54:415-20.
3. Dekker DL, Piziali RL, Dong E Jr. A system for ultrasonically imaging the human heart in three dimensions. Comput Biomed Res 1974;7:544-53.
4. Linker DT, Moritz WE, Pearlman AS. A new three-dimensional echocardiographic method of right ventricular volume measurement: in vitro validation. J Am Coll Cardiol 1986;8:101-6.
5. Matsumoto M, Matsuo H, Kitabatake A, et al. Three-dimensional echocardiograms and two-dimensional echocardiographic images at desired planes by a computerized system. Ultrasound Med Biol 1977;3:163-78.
6. von Ramm OT, Smith SW. Real time volumetric ultrasound imaging system. J Digital Imaging 1990;3:261-6.
7. Salgo IS. Three-dimensional echocardiographic technology. Cardiol Clin 2007;25:231-9.
8. Park SE, Shrout TR. Characteristics of relaxor-based piezoelectric single crystals for ultrasonic transducers. IEEE Trans. Ultrason Ferroelectr Freq Control 1997;44:1140-7.

9. Kuwata J, Uchino K, Nomura S. Dielectric and piezoelectric properties of 0.91Pb(Zn1/3Nb2/ O3-0.09PbTiO3 single crystals. Jpn J Appl Phys 1982;21:1298-302.
10. Gururaja TR, Panda RK, Chen J. Single crystal transducers for medical imaging applications. Ultrasonics Symposium Proc 1999;2:969-72.
11. Acar P, Abadir S, Paranon S, et al. Live 3D echocardiography with the pediatric matrix probe. Echocardiography 2007;24:750-5.
12. Simpson JM. Real-time three-dimensional echocardiography of congenital heart disease using a high frequency paediatric matrix transducer. Eur J Echocardiogr 2007 [Epub ahead of print].
13. Gopal AS, Chukwu EO, Iwuchukwu CJ, et al. Normal values of right ventricular size and function by real-time 3-dimensional echocardiography: comparison with cardiac magnetic resonance imaging. J Am Soc Echocardiogr 2007;20:445-55.
14. Niemann PS, Pinho L, Balbach T, et al. Anatomically oriented right ventricular volume measurements with dynamic three-dimensional echocardiography validated by 3-Tesla magnetic resonance imaging. J Am Coll Cardiol 2007;50:1668-76.
15. Salgo IS, Gorman JH 3rd, Gorman RC, et al. Effect of annular shape on leaflet curvature in reducing mitral leaflet stress. Circulation 2002;106:711-7.
16. Watanabe N, Ogasawara Y, Yamaura Y, et al. Mitral annulus flattens in ischemic mitral regurgitation: geometric differences between inferior and anterior myocardial infarction: a real-time 3-dimensional echocardio graphic study. Circulation 2005;112:I458-62.
17. Vogel M, Losch S. Dynamic three-dimensional echocardiography with a computed tomography imaging probe: initial clinical experience with transthoracic application in infants and children with congenital heart defects. Br Heart J 1994;71:462-7.
18. Vogel M, Ho SY, Anderson RH. Comparison of three dimensional echocardiographic findings with anatomical specimens of various congenitally malformed hearts. Br Heart J 1995;73: 566-70.
19. Vogel M, Ho SY, Buhlmeyer K, et al. Assessment of congenital heart defects by dynamic three-dimensional echocardiography: methods of data acquisition and clinical potential. Acta Paediatr Suppl 1995;410:34-9.
20. Espinola-Zavaleta N, Vargas-Barron J, Keirns C, et al. Three-dimensional echocardiography in congenital malformations of the mitral valve. J Am Soc Echocardiogr 2002;15:468-72.
21. Lu Q, Lu X, Xie M, et al. Real-time three-dimensional echocardiography in assessment of congenital double orifice mitral valve. J Huazhong Univ Sci Technolog Med Sci 2006;26:625-8.
22. Rawlins DB, Austin C, Simpson JM. Live three-dimensional paediatric intraoperative epicardial echocardiography as a guide to surgical repair of atrioventricular valves. Cardiol Young 2006;16:34-9.
23. Seliem MA, Fedec A, Szwast A, et al. Atrioventricular valve morphology and dynamics in congenital heart disease as imaged with real-time 3-dimensional matrix-array echocardiography: comparison with 2-dimensional imaging and surgical findings. J Am Soc Echocardiogr 2007;20:869-76.
24. Vettukattil JJ, Bharucha T, Anderson RH. Defining Ebstein's malformation using three-dimensional echocardiography. Interact Cardiovasc Thorac Surg 2007;6:685-90.
25. Hlavacek AM, Chessa K, Crawford FA, et al. Real-time three-dimensional echocardiography is useful in the evaluation of patients with atrioventricular septal defects. Echocardiography 2006;23:225-31.
26. Tantengco MV, Bates JR, Ryan T, et al. Dynamic three-dimensional echocardiographic reconstruction of congenital cardiac septation defects. Pediatr Cardiol 1997;18:184-90.
27. Cheng TO, Xie MX, Wang XF, et al. Real-time 3-dimensional echocardiography in assessing atrial and ventricular septal defects: an echo cardiographic-surgical correlative study. Am Heart J 2004;148:1091-5.
28. Mercer-Rosa L, Seliem MA, Fedec A, et al. Illustration of the additional value of real-time 3-dimensional echocardiography to conventional transthoracic and transesophageal 2-dimensional echocardiography in imaging muscular ventricular septal defects: Does this have any impact on individual patient treatment? J Am Soc Echocardiogr 2006;19:1511-9.
29. Hlavacek A, Lucas J, Baker H, et al. Feasibility and utility of three-dimensional color flow echocardiography of the aortic arch: the "echocardiographic angiogram". Echocardiography 2006;23:860-4.
30. Sadagopan SN, Veldtman GR, Sivaprakasam MC, et al. Correlations with operative anatomy of real time three-dimensional echocardio-graphic imaging of congenital aortic valvar stenosis. Cardiol Young 2006;16:490-4.
31. Bharucha T, Ho SY, Vettukattil JJ. Multiplanar review analysis of three-dimensional echocardiographic datasets gives new insights into the morphology of subaortic stenosis. Eur J Echo cardiogr 2008 [Epub ahead of print].
32. Baker GH, Pereira NL, Hlavacek AM, et al. Transthoracic real-time three-dimensional echocardiography in the diagnosis and description of noncompaction of ventricular myocardium. Echocardiography 2006;23:490-4.

33. Bu L, Munns S, Zhang H, et al. Rapid full volume data acquisition by real-time 3-dimensional echocardiography for assessment of left ventricular indexes in children: a validation study compared with magnetic resonance imaging. J Am Soc Echocardiogr 2005;18:299-305.
34. Baker GH, Flack EC, Hlavacek AM, et al. Variability and resource utilization of bedside three-dimensional echocardiographic quantitative measurements of left ventricular volume in congenital heart disease. Congenital Heart Dis 2006;1:318-23.
35. Mor-Avi V, Sugeng L, Weinert L, et al. Fast measurement of left ventricular mass with real-time three-dimensional echocardiography: comparison with magnetic resonance imaging. Circulation 2004;110:1814-8.
36. Pouleur AC, le Polain de Waroux JB, Pasquet A, et al. Assessment of left ventricular mass and volumes by three-dimensional echocardiography in patients with or without wall motion abnormalities: comparison against cine magnetic resonance imaging. Heart 2007 [Epub ahead of print].
37. Caiani EG, Corsi C, Zamorano J, et al. Improved semiautomated quantification of left ventricular volumes and ejection fraction using 3-dimensional echocardiography with a full matrix-array transducer: comparison with magnetic resonance imaging. J Am Soc Echocardiogr 2005;18:779-88.
38. Riehle TJ, Mahle WT, Parks WJ, et al. Real-time three-dimensional echocardiographic acquisition and quantification of left ventricular indices in children and young adults with congenital heart disease: comparison with magnetic resonance imaging. J Am Soc Echocardiogr 2008;21:78-83.
39. Kapetanakis S, Kearney MT, Siva A, et al. Real-time three-dimensional echocardiography: a novel technique to quantify global left ventricular mechanical dyssynchrony. Circulation 2005;112:992-1000.
40. Baker GH, Hlavacek AM, Chessa KS, et al. Left ventricular dysfunction is associated with intraventricular dyssynchrony by 3-dimensional echocardiography in children. J Am Soc Echocardiogr 2008;21:230-3.
41. Sugeng L, Weinert L, Lang RM. Real-time 3- dimensional color Doppler flow of mitral and tricuspid regurgitation: Feasibility and initial quantitative comparison with 2-dimensional methods. J Am Soc Echocardiogr 2007;20:1050-7.
42. Matsumura Y, Fukuda S, Tran H, et al. Geometry of the proximal isovelocity surface area in mitral regurgitation by 3 -dimensional color Doppler echocardiography: difference between functional mitral regurgitation and prolapse regurgitation. Am Heart J 2008; 155:231-8.
43. Sugeng L, Spencer KT, Mor-Avi V, et al. Dynamic three-dimensional color flow Doppler: an improved technique for the assessment of mitral regurgitation. Echocardiography 2003;20:265-73.
44. Pemberton J, Hui L, Young M, et al. Accuracy of 3-dimensional color Doppler-derived flow volumes with increasing image depth. J Ultrasound Med 2005;24:1109-15.
45. Pemberton J, Li X, Karamlou T, et al. The use of live three- dimensional Doppler echocardiography in the measurement of cardiac output: an in vivo animal study. J Am Coll Cardiol 2005;45:433-8.
46. Lodato JA, Weinert L, Baumann R, et al. Use of 3-dimensional color Doppler echocardiography to measure stroke volume in human beings: Comparison with thermodilution. J Am Soc Echocardiogr 2007;20:103-12.
47. Pemberton J, Ge S, Thiele K, et al. Real-time three-dimensional color Doppler echocardiography overcomes the inaccuracies of spectral Doppler for stroke volume calculation. J Am Soc Echocardiogr 2006;19:1403-10.
48. Scheurer M, Bandisode V, Ruff P, et al. Early experience with real-time three-dimensional echocardio-graphic guidance of right ventricular biopsy in children. Echocardiography 2006;23:45-9.
49. Suematsu Y, Martinez JF, Wolf BK, et al. Three-dimensional echo-guided beating heart surgery without cardiopulmonary bypass: atrial septal defect closure in a swine model. J Thorac Cardiovasc Surg 2005;130:1348-57.
50. Suematsu Y, Marx GR, Stoll JA, et al. Three-dimensional echocardiography-guided beating-heart surgery without cardiopulmonary bypass: a feasibility study. J Thorac Cardiovasc Surg 2004;128:579-87.
51. Suematsu Y, Marx GR, Triedman JK, et al. Three-dimensional echocardiography-guided atrial septectomy: an experimental study. J Thorac Cardiovasc Surg 2004;128:53-9.
52. Vasilyev NV, Martinez JF, Freudenthal FP, et al. Three-dimensional echo and videocardioscopy-guided atrial septal defect closure. Ann Thorac Surg 2006;82:1322-6.
53. Baker GH, Shirali GS, Bandisode V. Transseptal left heart catheterization for a patient with a prosthetic mitral valve using live three-dimensional transesophageal echocardiography. Pediatr Cardiol 2007 [Epub ahead of print].
54. Jenkins C, Monaghan M, Shirali G, et al. An intensive interactive course for 3D echocardiography: Is "Crop Till You Drop" an effective learning strategy? Eur J Echocardiogr 2007 [Epub ahead of print].

CHAPTER 8

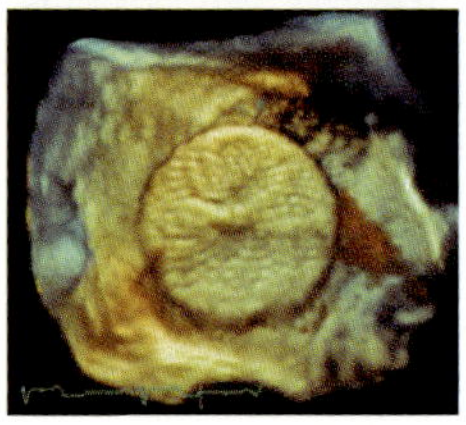

Transesophageal 3D Echocardiography for Device Closure of Atrial Septal Defects

Balu Vaidyanathan, John M Simpson, Raman Krishna Kumar

Transcatheter closure is an effective alternative to surgery in most patients with atrial septal defects (ASDs) of the secundum type.[1,2] Factors that decide suitability for transcatheter closure include size of the defect and presence of adequate tissue rims around the defect.[3] Accurate imaging of the anatomic features of the ASD is critical for case selection, planning, and guidance during the procedure. This is accomplished using 2-dimensional (2D) and 3-dimensional (3D)

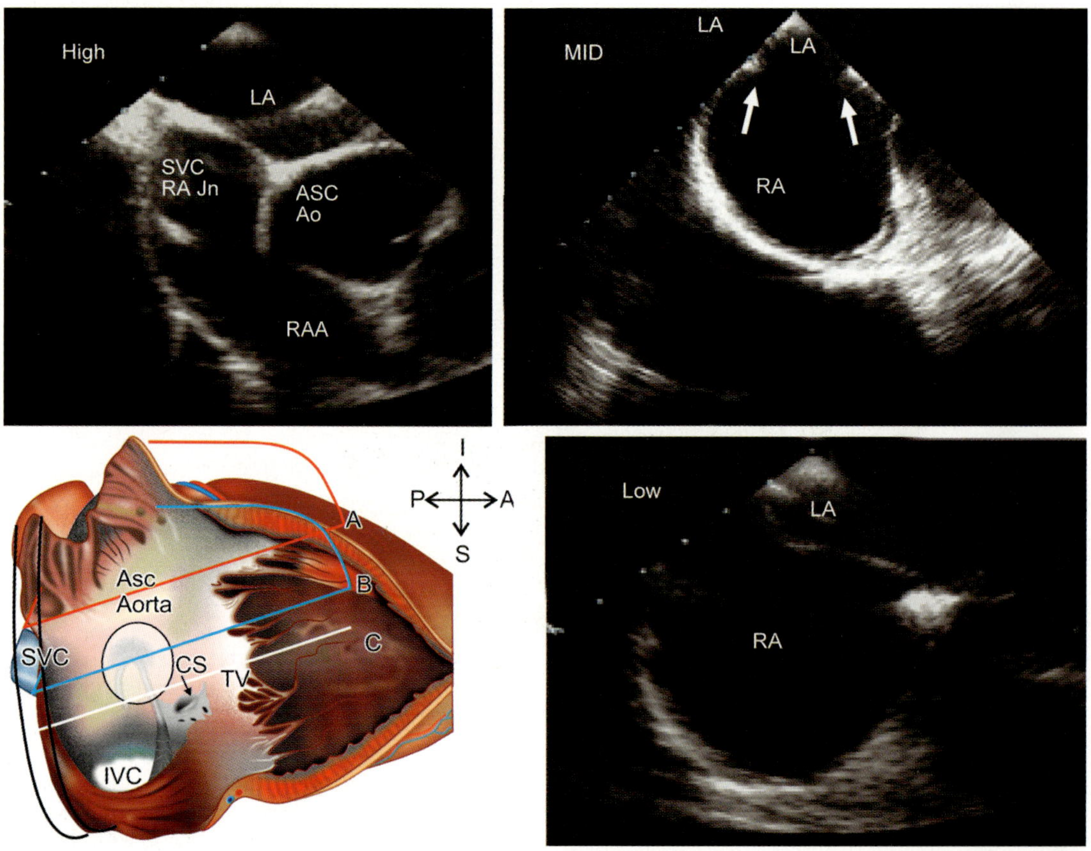

Figure 1: TEE at 0° to evaluate the posterior and anterior rims of the defect: The transesophageal echocardiography (TEE) probe is at the mid-lower esophageal level. The posterior and the mitral rims are best evaluated in this view. Rotating the probe to 30° to 40° towards the left will best profile the aortic (Ao) rim. The margins are evaluated by carefully moving the probe in and out and obtaining sections at various levels. In the highest plane. (A) The superior venacaval (SVC)-right atrial junction and the ascending (Asc) aorta are seen; the atrial septum is visualized as intact. At the mid-level. (B) The septum breaks and the margins of the atrial septal defects (ASD) (arrows) are clearly seen. At the level of the atrioventricular valves. (C) The septum forms once again. This suggests that the ASD is likely to have adequate margins for catheter closure. CS = coronary sinus; IVC = inferior venacaval; Jn = junction; LA = left atrium; RA = right atrium; RAA = right atrial appendage; TV = tricuspid valve

echocardiography and of late, intracardiac echocardiography (ICE). This review focuses on comprehensive imaging through transesophageal echocardiography (TEE) for transcatheter closure of ASDs (Figures 1 and 2).

ANATOMY OF THE ASD: NOMENCLATURE OF THE RIMS/MARGINS

Conventionally, the rims of a secundum ASD are labeled as aortic (superoanterior), atrioventricular (AV) valve (mitral or inferoanterior), superior venacaval (SVC or supero-posterior), inferior venacaval (IVC or inferoposterior), and posterior (from the posterior free wall of the atria). By conventional definition, a margin >5 mm is considered to be adequate.[3] Podnar et al[4] defined 10 morphological variations of defects, the most common type being the defect with deficient aortic rim (42.1%). The other variants included central defects (24.2%), deficient inferoposterior rim (12.1%), perforated aneurysm of the septum (7.9%), multiple defects (7.3%), combined deficiency of mitral and aortic rims (4.1%), deficient SVC rim (1%), and deficient coronary sinus rim (1%) (Figures 3 and 4).

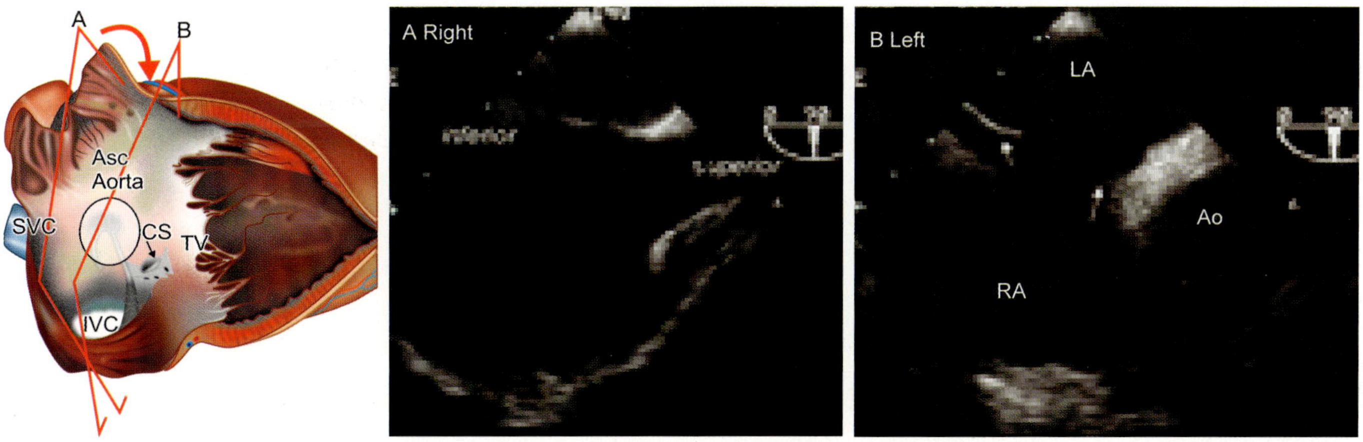

Figure 2: TEE at 90° to evaluate the SVC and IVC rims: This view is best for evaluating the SVC and IVC rims. The margins are evaluated by rotating the probe while keeping it at more or less the same level. Here the defect is seen with the probe rotated leftward (B, margins of the ASD shown by the **arrows**), while septum is seen to form when the probe is rotated to the right (A). The 45°-view is helpful in assessing the posterior and the aortic rims and often helps to determine the maximum size of the defect. Abbreviations are as in Figure 1.

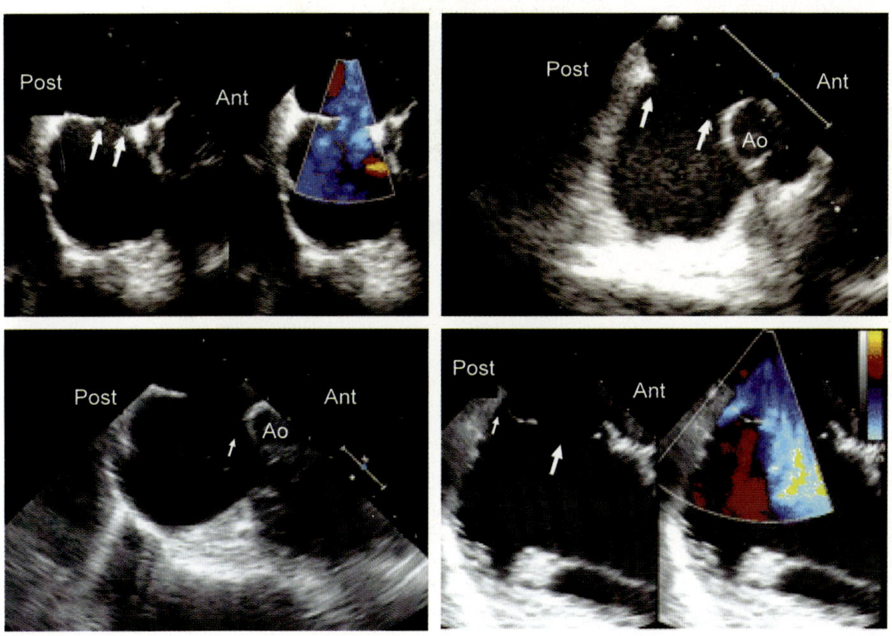

Figure 3: Different morphological variations of ASD as Demonstrated Using TEE: Panel A shows a centrally located ASD imaged at 0°; the posterior (Post) and the anterior (Ant) margins are clearly demonstrated **(arrows)**. **Panel B** shows an ASD with deficient Ao margin **(arrow)**. Both of these types of ASDs can be easily closed using the transcatheter technique (4). **Panel C** shows a large ASD with deficient posterior and Ao margins **(arrows)**. This type of ASD is technically challenging for device closure and requires specialized imaging and deployment techniques.[5] **Panel D** shows multiple ASDs; there is a larger anterior defect **(block arrow)** and a smaller posterior defect **(thin arrow)**. This type of ASD is amenable for device closure, often with a single device. Abbreviations are as in Figure 1.

SPECIAL TEE VIEWS FOR IMAGING THE INFEROPOSTERIOR RIM

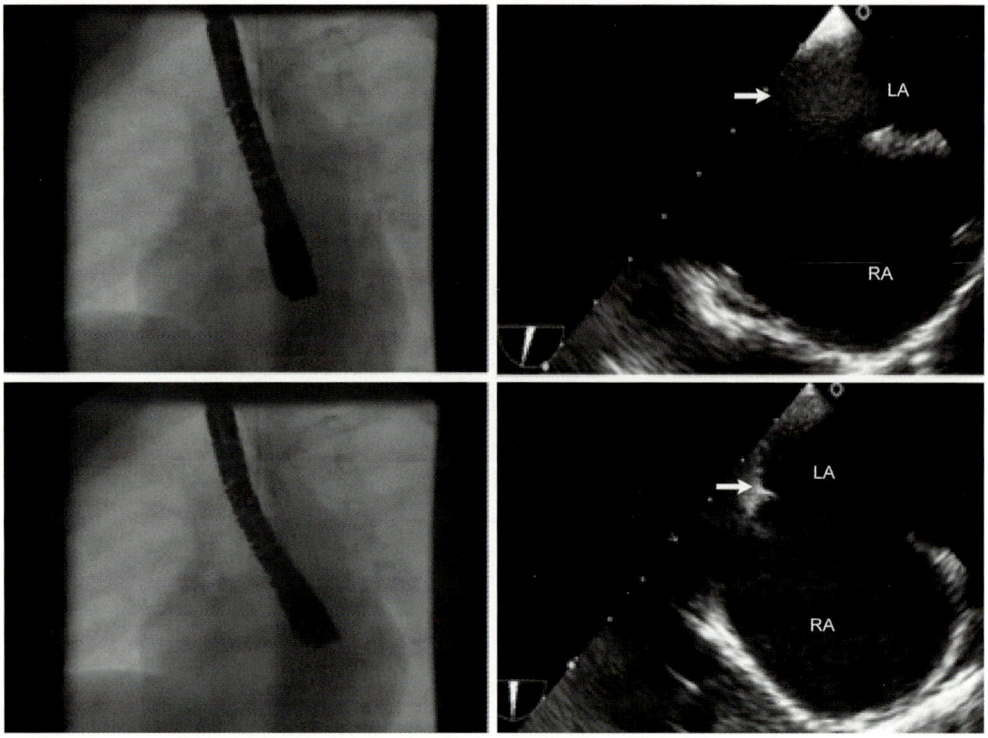

Figure 4: **Retroflexed TEE view for imaging the inferoposterior rim:** The IVC rim cannot be profiled well through conventional TEE techniques because of the proximity of the IVC to the lower esophagus. **Panel A** demonstrates the fluoroscopic image of the TEE probe by using the conventional method. **Panel B** depicts the TEE images thus obtained. The inferoposterior rim **(arrow)** is not clearly profiled. **Panel C** demonstrates the retroflexed TEE probe position on fluoroscopy. The TEE probe is advanced into the stomach, retroflexed, and slowly withdrawn to lower esophagus. Imaging is performed in the long axis at 70° to 90°. The probe along with the lower esophagus moves away from the IVC-right atrial junction and the ultrasound beam is directed perpendicular to the IVC rim thus profiling the IVC rim **(arrow)** clearly **(D)**.[5] Abbreviations are as in Figure 1.

3D ECHOCARDIOGRAPHY

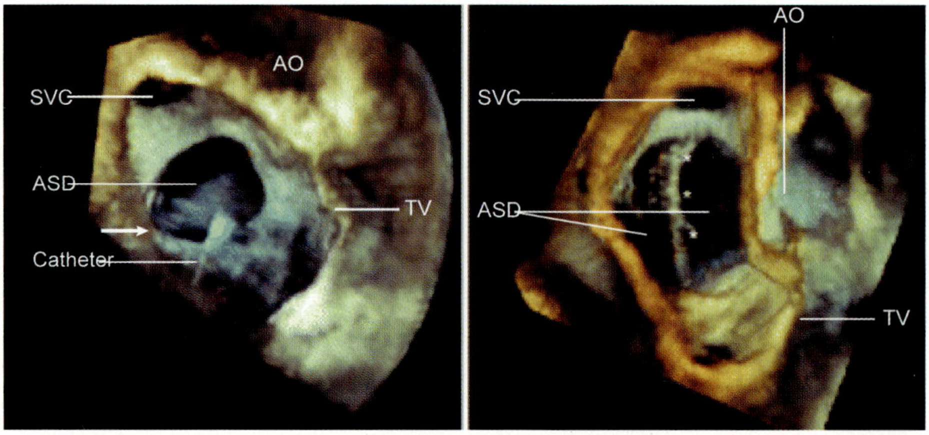

Figure 5: **3D echocardiography for evaluation of ASD size and margins:** This is performed using "matrix" transducers which allow acquisition of a pyramid-shaped volume of echocardiographic data. To achieve the highest resolution of the atrial septum and adjacent structures, a "full-volume" 3 dimensional (3D) dataset is obtained over 4 to 7 cardiac cycles. For transthoracic 3D images, the subcostal view is the preferred view because its projection is en face to the atrial septum; in patients with suboptimal windows the low parasternal 4-chamber view may be used. 3D TEE overcomes the limitation of poor acoustic windows in adult patients (>25 kg) **(A and B)**. Real-time 3D imaging demonstrates the changing shape of the ASD **(Online Video 3)** during a cardiac cycle, with maximum size in diastole.[6] **Panel A** shows an en face 3D reconstruction of a secundum ASD with a relatively deficient IVC and posterior rim **(arrow). Panel B** demonstrates multiple ASDs with the thin atrial septum **(*)** separating the 2 defects. Abbreviations are as in Figure 1.

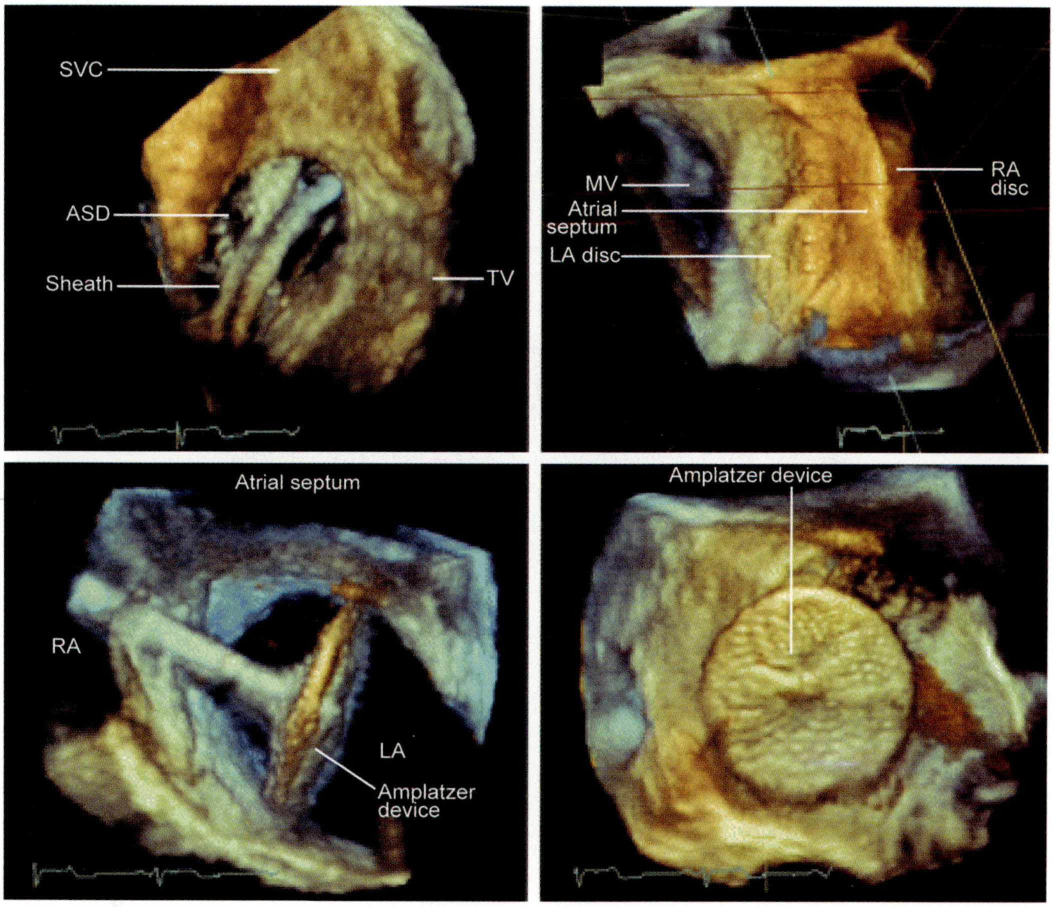

Figure 6: 3D TEE to guide deployment and assess device position during the procedure, "live 3D" or a "3D zoom" mode is used to observe the position of guidewires, sheaths, and devices in real time. **Panel A** depicts a 3D image of the ASD from the right atrial side demonstrating the delivery sheath being positioned through the defect. 3D echocardiography is particularly helpful in patients with multiple ASDs to ensure placement of the delivery sheath through the bigger defect. 3D echocardiography can be potentially helpful in patients with difficult ASDs by demonstrating the alignment of the disks against the septum during deployment.[7] **Panel B** demonstrates the deployment of the LA disk which is still attached to the deployment catheter. The LA disk is fully expanded and is seen to align well against the atrial septum. **Panel C** demonstrates the ASD device post-deployment; the device is well aligned against the septum and both the discs are well visualized on either side. **Panel D** illustrates an en face reconstruction of the Amplatzer device from the LA side post-deployment. The device is seen snugly fitting to the ASD margins **(Online Video 6).**

2D TEE

For a comprehensive evaluation of the ASD, TEE is performed in 3 different planes: transverse (0°), longitudinal (90°), and at 45°.

MV = mitral valve; other abbreviations as in Figure 1.

Echocardiography plays a critical role for patient selection, guidance, and post-deployment evaluation for transcatheter closure of ASDs. Understanding the echoanatomic corelation by transeso phageal echocardiography is perhaps the most essential requisite to ensure a successful procedure. 3D echocardiography is likely to further this understanding in the future especially in difficult cases like multiple defects and defects with deficient margins (Figures 5 and 6).

Address for correspondence: Dr Raman Krishna Kumar, Pediatric Cardiology, Amrita Institute of Medical Sciences, AIMS Ponekkara PO, Kochi, Kerala 682 041, India (Email: rkrishnakumar@aims.amrita.edu).

REFERENCES

1. Harper RW, Mottram PM, McGaw DJ. Closure of secundum atrial septal defects with the Amplatzer septal occluder device: techniques and problems Catheter Cardiovasc Interv 2002;57:508-24. [CrossRef][Web of Science][Medline]
2. Butera G, Romagnoli E, Carminati M, et al. Treatment of isolated secundum atrial septal defects: impact of age and defect morphology in 1013 consecutive patients Am Heart J 2008;156:706-12.[CrossRef][Web of Science][Medline]
3. Cooke JC, Gelman JS, Harper RW. Echocardiologist's role in the deployment of the Amplatzer septal occlude device in adults J Am Soc Echocardiogr 2001;14:588-94. [CrossRef] [Web of Science][Medline]
4. Podnar T, Martanovic P, Gavora P, Masura J. Morphological variations of secundum-type atrial septal defects: feasibility for percutaneous closure using Amplatzer septal occluders Catheter Cardiovasc Interv 2001;53:386-91. [CrossRef][Web of Science] [Medline]
5. Remadevi KS, Francis E, Kumar RK. Catheter closure of atrial septal defects with deficient inferior vena cava rim under transesophageal echo guidance Catheter Cardiovasc Interv 2009;73:90-6. [CrossRef][Web of Science][Medline]
6. Van den Bosch AE, Harkel DJT, McGhie JS, et al. Characterization of atrial septal defect assessed by real time 3 dimensional echocardiography J Am Soc Echocardiogr 2006;19:815-21. [CrossRef][Web of Science][Medline]
7. Balzer J, Kelm M, Kuhl HP. Real-time three-dimensional transoesophageal echocardiography for guidance of non-coronary interventions in the catheter laboratory Eur J Echocardiogr 2009;108:341-9. [Abstract/Free Full Text]

CHAPTER 9

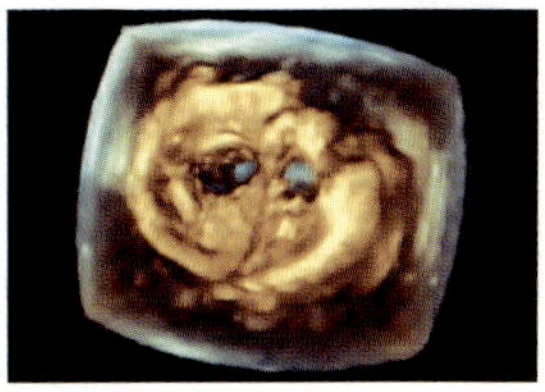

TEE Guided Interventions and Advantages of 3D TEE

V Amuthan, P Ashok Kumar

INTRODUCTION

Traditionally, percutaneous cardiovascular interventions have predominantly used angiographic and fluoroscopic guidance, which is limited when interventions involve the myocardium, pericardium, and cardiac valves. Echocardiography has emerged as an effective alternative imaging modality in the cardiac catheterization lab. A major advantage of echocardiography over other advanced imaging modalities (magnetic resonance imaging, computed tomographic angiography) is that echocardiography is mobile and real time. Echocardiograms can be recorded at the bedside, in the cardiac catheterization laboratory, in the cardiovascular intensive care unit, in the emergency room—indeed, any place that can accommodate a wheeled cart. This tremendous advantage allows for the performance of imaging immediately before, during, and after various procedures involving interventions.

PROCEDURES PERFORMED UNDER ECHOCARDIOGRAPHIC GUIDANCE

Echocardiographic guidance is routinely sought for during the following procedures,

1. Transatrial septal catheterization, Chapter 9 Video 1
2. Percutaneous transvenous balloon valvuloplasty, Chapter 9 Video 2 showing Inoue Balloon across Mitral valve
3. Catheter closure of atrial septal defects (ASDs) and patent foramen ovale (PFO), Chapter 9 Video 3
4. Pericardiocentesis,
5. Myocardial biopsy,
6. Alcohol septal ablation for hypertrophic cardiomyopathy, and
7. Cardiac electrophysiology.

Recently, complex mitral valve repairs, left atrial appendage (LAA) occlusion devices, percutaneous aortic valve replacement and cardiac resynchronization therapy procedures also demand echo guidance for their successful performance.[1]

GENERAL IMAGING CONSIDERATIONS

TRANSTHORACIC ECHOCARDIOGRAPHY (TTE)

TTE is widely available and portable and offers excellent image quality; as such, it has been used widely in guiding percutaneous noncoronary interventional and electrophysiologic procedures. Most currently available ultrasound systems, including handheld and portable ultrasound systems, offer sufficient 2-dimensional (2D) and Doppler capabilities to guide a variety of interventions, such as echocardiography guided pericardiocentesis, alcohol septal ablation for hypertrophic cardiomyopathy, percutaneous balloon mitral valvuloplasty (PTMC), and myocardial biopsy. The advent of Doppler tissue imaging has made TTE essential in the optimization of biventricular pacemakers.

TRANSESOPHAGEAL ECHOCARDIOGRAPHY (TEE)

TEE has been widely used as an alternative to TTE in guiding complex procedures. TEE offers superior image resolution to TTE and can be used to monitor a variety of interventions, such as percutaneous transcatheter closure (PTC) of septal defects, PTMC, transseptal catheterization, and many others. Compared with TTE, it excels at assessing intraprocedural anatomy and physiology, monitoring catheter position and contact, and excluding thrombus, pericardial effusion, and other complications.

ECHOCARDIOGRAPHY IN TRANSSEPTAL CATHETERIZATION

Transseptal catheterization is performed when procedural access to the left atrium is required and is used for PTMC, anterograde aortic balloon valvuloplasty, radiofrequency ablation of AF and other left-sided arrhythmias, transseptal PFO closure, the placement of percutaneous left ventricular assist device cannulas in the left atrium, balloon or blade atrial septostomy, the measurement of complex hemodynamics (such as evaluation of a mechanical aortic valve prosthesis or critical aortic stenosis in which the valve itself cannot be crossed), and, most recently, investigational applications such as the placement of LAA occlusion devices and percutaneous mitral valve repair.

Transesophageal echo offers potential advantages over traditional anatomic and fluoroscopic guidance.[2] Anatomic variability in the position and orientation of the fossa ovalis and its surrounding structures may present specific challenges to even those interventional cardiologists with significant transseptal experience, and imaging offers increased safety, with a lower risk for cannulating other spaces adjacent to the fossa. Inadvertent puncture of the intrapericardial aorta is a serious complication of transseptal catheterization, and echocardiographic imaging reduces this risk. Similarly, imaging may decrease the time required for the transseptal puncture to be performed and minimizes the fluoroscopy time required for the procedure.

TEE provides the ability to choose the exact site of transseptal puncture, which is important in performing advanced mitral valve interventions for mitral regurgitation (MR) because the catheters are more difficult to manipulate and position if the transseptal crossing point is too close to the plane of the mitral valve orifice. Chapter 9 Video 4 Passing of LA wire after Trans septal puncture.

ECHOCARDIOGRAPHIC GUIDANCE OF PERCUTANEOUS TRANSVENOUS MITRAL COMMISUROTOMY

PTMC is performed with fluoroscopic guidance alone at many centers, but radiographic anatomic landmarks can mislead even experienced operators. Kronzon et al recommended 2D TTE (in the apical 4-chamber and parasternal short-axis views) as a useful adjunct to fluoroscopy during transseptal cardiac catheterization during PTMC.[3] Pandian et al advocated the use of subcostal views to assist PTMC as well.[4] Disadvantages of TTE include that it interrupts the flow of the procedure, potentially interferes with sterile technique, and provides inadequate imaging in some patients.

TEE is an alternative to TTE for guiding PTMC. TEE can be used for patient selection and for all aspects of online procedural guidance (Figure 1 and Chapter 9 video 5). It is used to guide the transseptal catheterization and is generally superior to TTE in this regard. TEE is also superior to TTE when it is used to exclude left atrial and LAA thrombus, and it facilitates wire and balloon position before and during inflation. TEE is used to measure transmitral gradients and mitral valve area and to assess the degree of MR immediately after each balloon inflation. Finally, TEE can be used to look for complications of PTMC, such as severe MR, pericardial effusion or tamponade, dislodgement of thrombus, and residual ASD.

IMMEDIATE ASSESSMENT OF RESULTS

Online echocardiography during the procedure is ideally suited for the immediate assessment of the results of PTMC. The adequacy of valvulotomy can be determined by evaluating the maximal mitral leaflet separation and by continuous-wave Doppler determination of the mean mitral gradient and mitral valve area (Figures 2 and 3). With TEE in addition, the pulmonary venous flow profile can be assessed, with a more rapid diastolic deceleration expected after successful PTMC. Finally, new or worsening MR is sought by color Doppler. Decisions about the adequacy of the procedure versus the need for further dilation should be made on the basis of both echocardiographic and hemodynamic data.

EARLY DETECTION OF COMPLICATIONS

Although uncommon, serious complications do occur with PTMC. The majority of these (e.g. the development of severe MR, cardiac perforation and tamponade, ASDs) can be identified accurately and quickly by online echocardiography during the procedure. An increase in the degree of MR occurs in approximately half of patients after PTMC.[5] In most, this increase is mild, but the reported incidence of the development of severe MR is 1% to 6%.[5] Acute, severe

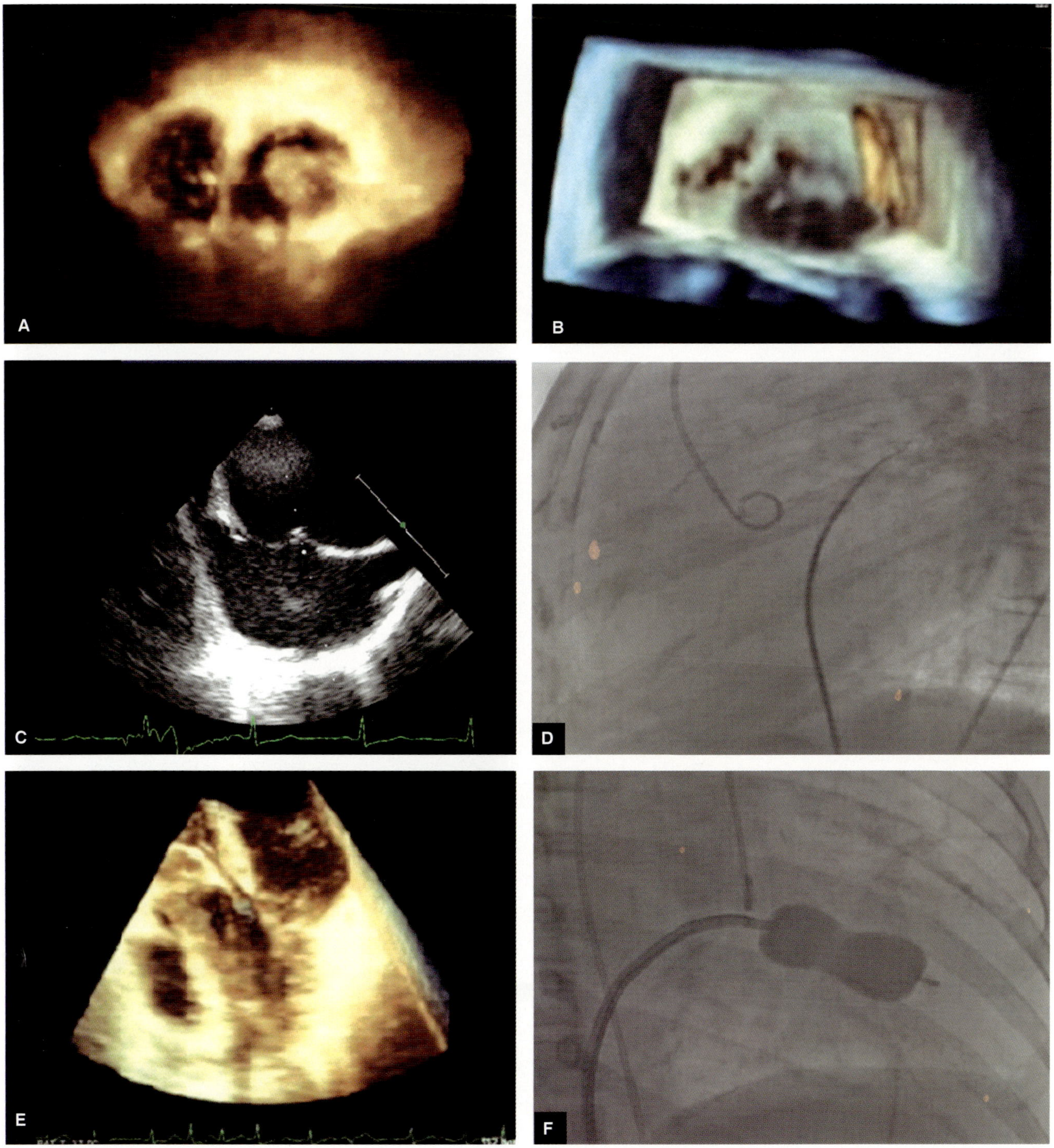

Figure 1: A case of Mitral Stenosis. (A) and (B) showing the valve as seen from the LA aspect before and after PTMC. (C) and (D) showing the septal puncture by echo (C) and fluoroscopy (D). (E) and (F) showing the balloon dilatation by 3D TEE (E) and fluoroscopy (F)

MR may be caused by tear or rupture of the mitral leaflets, by ruptured chordae tendineae, or rarely by avulsion of a papillary muscle.[6] Each of these can be detected readily by echocardiography, particularly by TEE. Moreover, the presence and severity of MR can be determined without the need for ventriculography. The incidence of cardiac

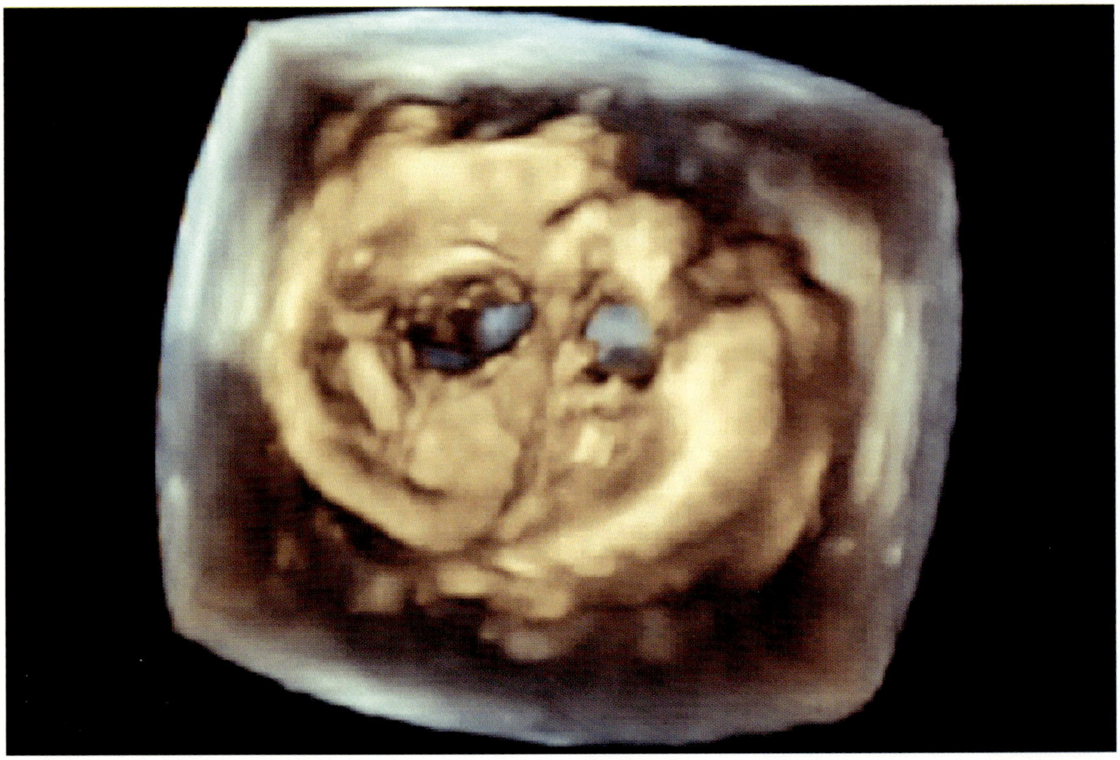

Figure 2: Mitral valve in a patient with mitral stenosis after PTMC

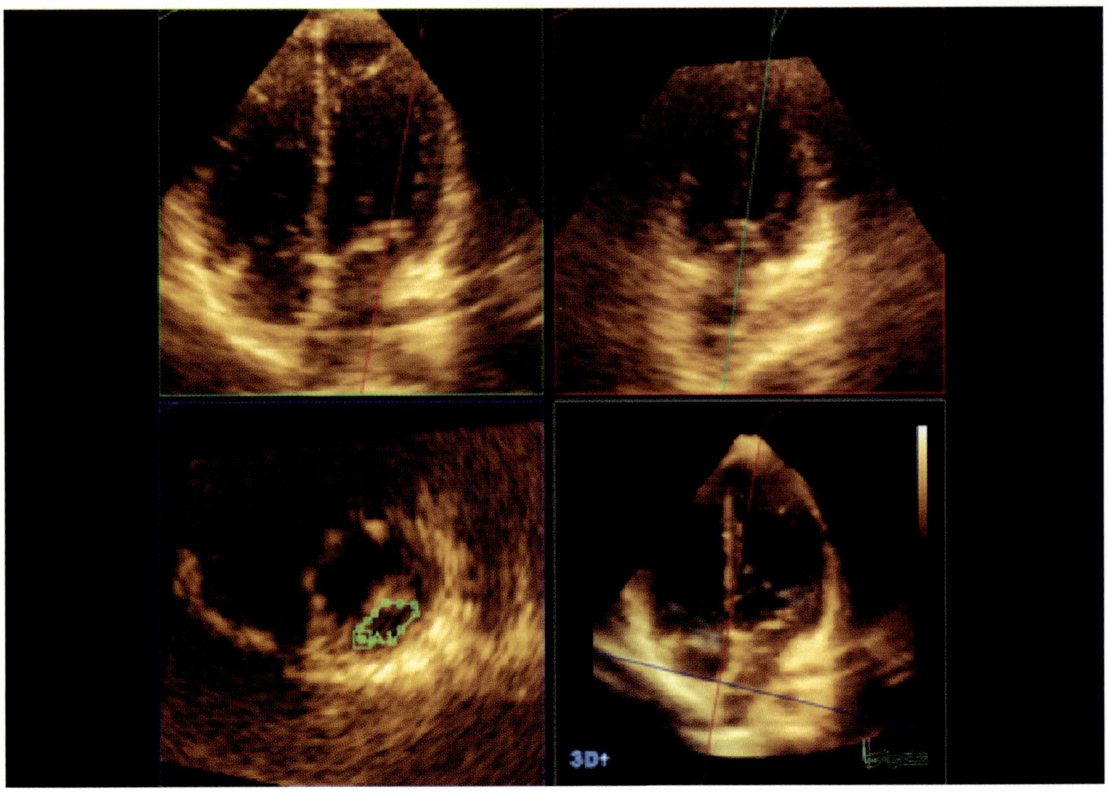

Figure 3: Post-PTMC mitral valve area measurement

tamponade during PTMC has been reported to be between 0% and 9%. Perforation of the atrial free wall at the time of transseptal puncture is the most common cause of bleeding into the pericardial space. Echocardiographic detection of such fluid is immediate and permits rapid pericardiocentesis before major hemodynamic compromise occurs. Perforation of the left ventricle, especially with the double-balloon technique, has also been reported. Online TEE can lead to rapid detection and treatment of this potentially life threatening complication. The reported incidence of ASD resulting from PTMC is highly variable depending on the technique used for its detection TTE can detect an atrial shunt after PTMC in 15% to 60% of patients. TEE, a more sensitive technique, has been reported to detect shunts in as many as 90% of patients.

EFFECT ON OUTCOMES

The use of echocardiographic guidance during the procedure may improve the procedural success and complication rates.[7] Online imaging can provide more precise targeting of the transseptal needle toward the fossa ovalis region of the atrial septum, thereby minimizing the likelihood of perforation. In addition, imaging not only has the potential to reduce the risk for procedural complications but may also allow immediate identification of these complications should they occur, permitting more prompt correction. Moreover, echocardiographic guidance may reduce procedural and fluoroscopic time. Park et al[8] evaluated fluoroscopic guidance only (n = 64) in patients who underwent PTMC with online transesophageal echocardiographic guidance (n = 70). The procedural time was significantly shorter in the latter group (99 6 48 vs 64 6 22 minutes; P < .0001). The average fluoroscopic time was also shorter in the TEE-guided group (306 17 vs 19 6 15 minutes), but this was not statistically significant (P = .25). Echocardiographic guidance may also reduce the risk for worsening MR as a result of the better assessment of the number of balloon inflations required and better positioning of the balloon catheter. Further studies are required to validate the incremental safety and efficacy of echocardiographic guidance to supplement or replace fluoroscopic guidance of PTMC.

SUMMARY GUIDELINES[1]

Echocardiography provides significant benefit in percutaneous balloon valvuloplasty for mitral stenosis and is recommended for the assessment of patient selection and to assess the adequacy of results. Online intraprocedural echocardiography offers significant advantages compared with fluoroscopic guidance, in monitoring procedural efficacy and monitoring for complications. TEE can also be used to guide the procedure. TTE is recommended for procedural guidance, monitoring for complications, and to assess the adequacy of results, when preprocedural TEE has already been performed. ICE can be used for procedural guidance and provides imaging that is comparable with TEE.

ADVANTAGES OF 3D TEE[9]

Although 2-dimensional echocardiography remains the standard imaging modality for evaluating mitral stenosis, the advent of 3-dimensional (3D) transthoracic echocardiography (TTE) and 3D transesophageal echocardiography (TEE) harbor the potential to revolutionize the noninvasive evaluation and invasive management (i.e. PTMC) of severe mitral stenosis. Before the development of real-time 3-dimensional (RT3D) imaging, the use of 3D echocardiography in evaluating mitral stenosis was limited to offline reconstruction of gated 3D images acquired using 2-dimensional echocardiography before PTMC. Although offline reconstruction helped to clarify the presence and extent of commissural fusion, it could be used for neither procedural guidance nor as a mechanism for immediate feedback on procedural results.

After the introduction of RT3D TTE in 2002, it became obvious that this technological advancement would serve as a useful tool to enhance our understanding and evaluation of mitral commissural fusion by providing "depth" to the mitral valve through the application of the "elevation" dimension (i.e. the third dimension). Furthermore, as opposed to the gated technique, RT3D imaging allowed visualization of the mitral valve throughout an unlimited number of cardiac cycles. Finally, the same evaluation could be performed before and after PTMC as well as during the balloon inflation. Indeed, using the technology during PTMC procedures, we noted several dramatic demonstrations of commissural splitting shown with pre and post-procedure RT3D TTE. The advent of RT3D TEE in November 2007, however, represented the next frontier in the evaluation of mitral stenosis and allowed for optimal 3D imaging of the mitral commissures in virtually all patients. As a result, we have now transitioned to routinely using RT3D TEE to both preprocedurally evaluate mitral stenosis (i.e. assessing commissural fusion) and assess the immediate results (i.e. assessing CO) of PTMC. Additonally, the enhanced imaging provided by RT3D TEE has provided an improved confidence in adopting the approach to PTMC of proceeding with increased Inoue balloon inflations until one or both commissures are split, while exercising caution to stop earlier should progressive mitral regurgitation develop. In summary, we agree with Messika-Zeitoun et al[10] that 3D echocardiography, but particularly RT3D TEE, offers tremendous potential in assessing commissural fusion in mitral stenosis and CO after PTMC, although further evaluation of this novel imaging modality is clearly needed before widespread adoption is achieved. Nonetheless, our positive experiences in using RT3D echocardiography in both the evaluation and the treatment of mitral stenosis have led to our laboratory incorporating it as a mainstay in the evaluation and percutaneous treatment of severe mitral stenosis.

ECHOCARDIOGRAPHIC GUIDANCE OF ATRIAL SEPTAL DEFECT AND PATENT FORAMEN OVALE CLOSURE

Percutaneous transcatheter closure of ASDs and PFO is an increasingly attractive alternative to surgical repair. These procedures are widely performed for hemodynamically significant left-to-right shunting, to prevent recurrent paradoxical embolism, and for the platypnea- orthodeoxia syndrome.

TEE is used to evaluate and guide the percutaneous closure of PFOs and ASDs. TTE has the advantage of offering multiple planes to evaluate the device and atrial septum, but it has limited ability to interrogate the lower rim of atrial septal tissue above the inferior vena cava after device placement, because the device interferes with imaging in virtually all planes. In addition, because the septum is relatively far from the transducer, color imaging is suboptimal in larger patients. Some centers, however, use TTE for monitoring in all patients. Transesophageal echocardiographic guidance has been described extensively in adult patients and offers the advantages of providing real-time, highly detailed imaging of the interatrial septum, surrounding structures, catheters, and closure device.

3D TEE GUIDED DEVICE CLOSURE

The use of percutaneously delivered devices for ASD or PFO repair is increasing. Three-dimensional imaging allows for accurate anatomic assessment before the procedure and can localize the closure device during the procedure in relation to other cardiac structures, potentially enhancing success and possibly decreasing the complication rate[11] (Figures 4 and 5). In 40 of 41 patients (98%) undergoing device ASD closure, 3D images of defects were obtained, and these images more accurately assessed ASD size (using balloon sizing as the "gold standard") than did 2D TEE. Additionally, device position was more accurately assessed with 3D imaging.[12,13] Real-time 3D echocardiography has also been used for accurate assessment of the morphology and efficacy of transcatheter devices used for ASD and PFO closure. See also Chapter 9 Video 6.

OTHER RARE CONGENITAL HEART DISEASES

3D echocardiography aids in the understanding of the anatomy of rare congenital heart diseases like Coronary AV fistulas and aid in their percutaneous management (Figure 6). Coil/Device closure for such cases simplifies the management options. The preprocedure assessment of the site of origin and exit by echocardiography is key to the success of the procedure.

ECHOCARDIOGRAPHIC GUIDANCE OF ALCOHOL SEPTAL ABLATION FOR HYPERTROPHIC OBSTRUCTIVE CARDIOMYOPATHY

Alcohol septal ablation involves the introduction of alcohol into a target septal perforator branch of the left anterior descending coronary artery for the purpose of producing a myocardial infarction within the proximal ventricular septum.

Since the introduction of this procedure by Sigwart, a number of other groups have applied and modified this technique with good results.[14] Perhaps the most important modification has been the use of myocardial contrast echocardiography to delineate the vascular distribution of the individual septal perforator branches of the left anterior descending artery. In fact, the use of contrast echocardiography is paramount to the success of this procedure.[15]

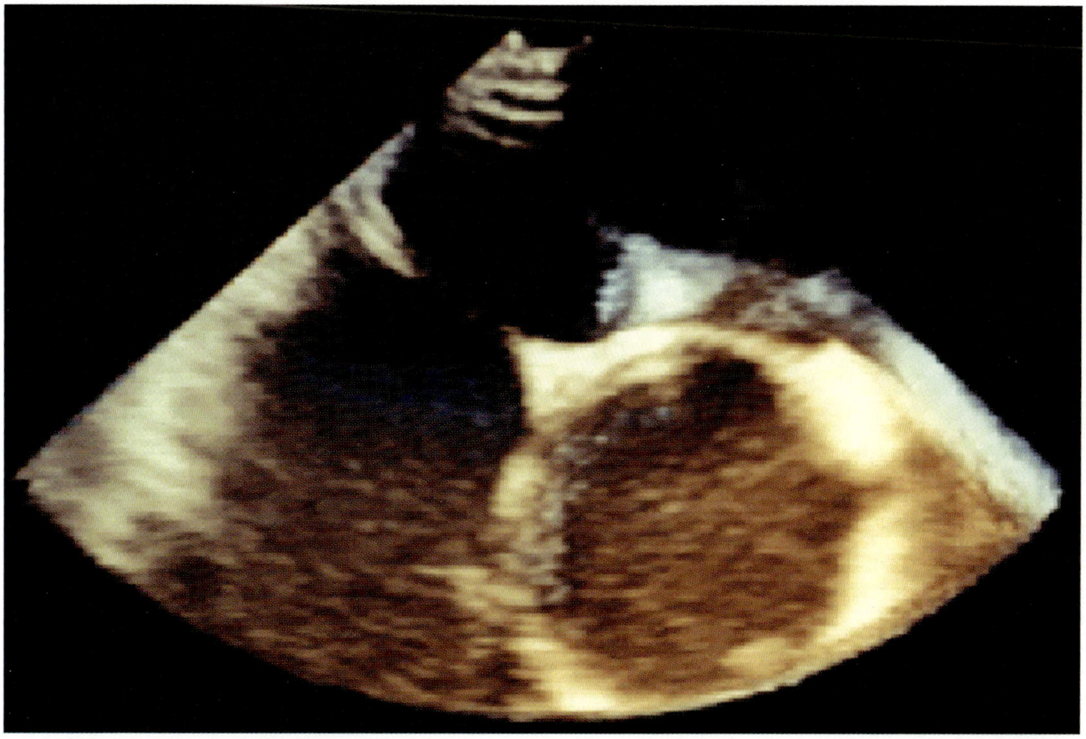

Figure 4: 3D TEE showing the aortic rim and the posterior rim of ASD

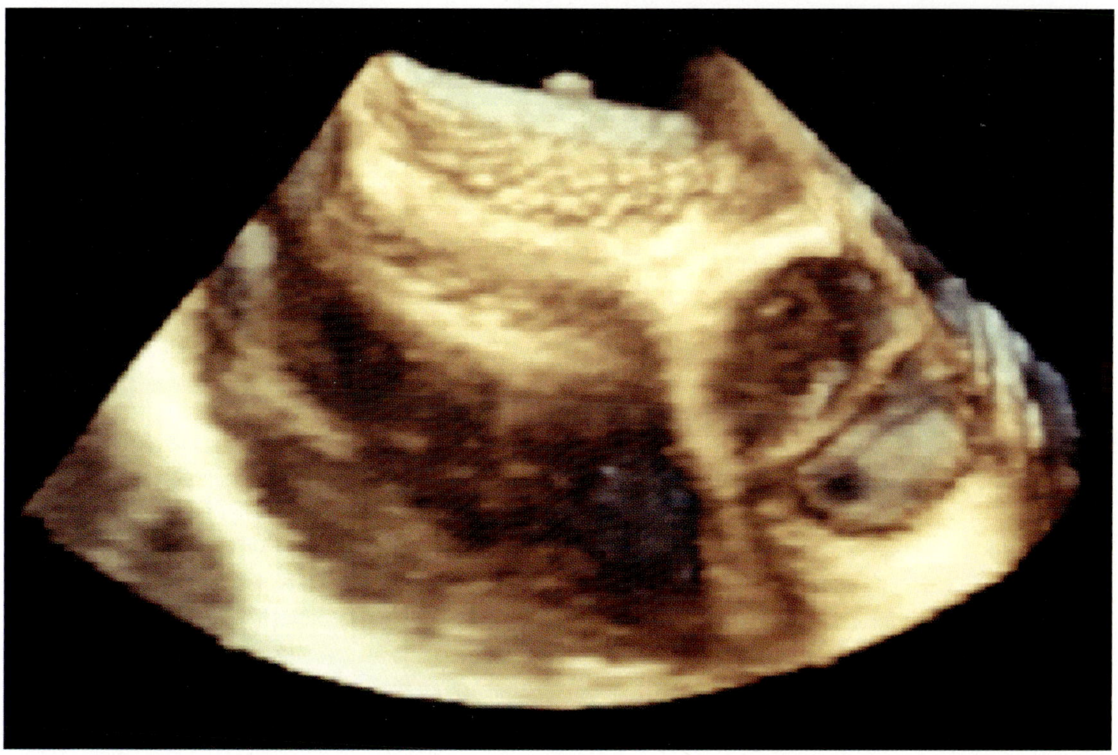

Figure 5: 3D TEE showing the ASD device in situ across the IAS

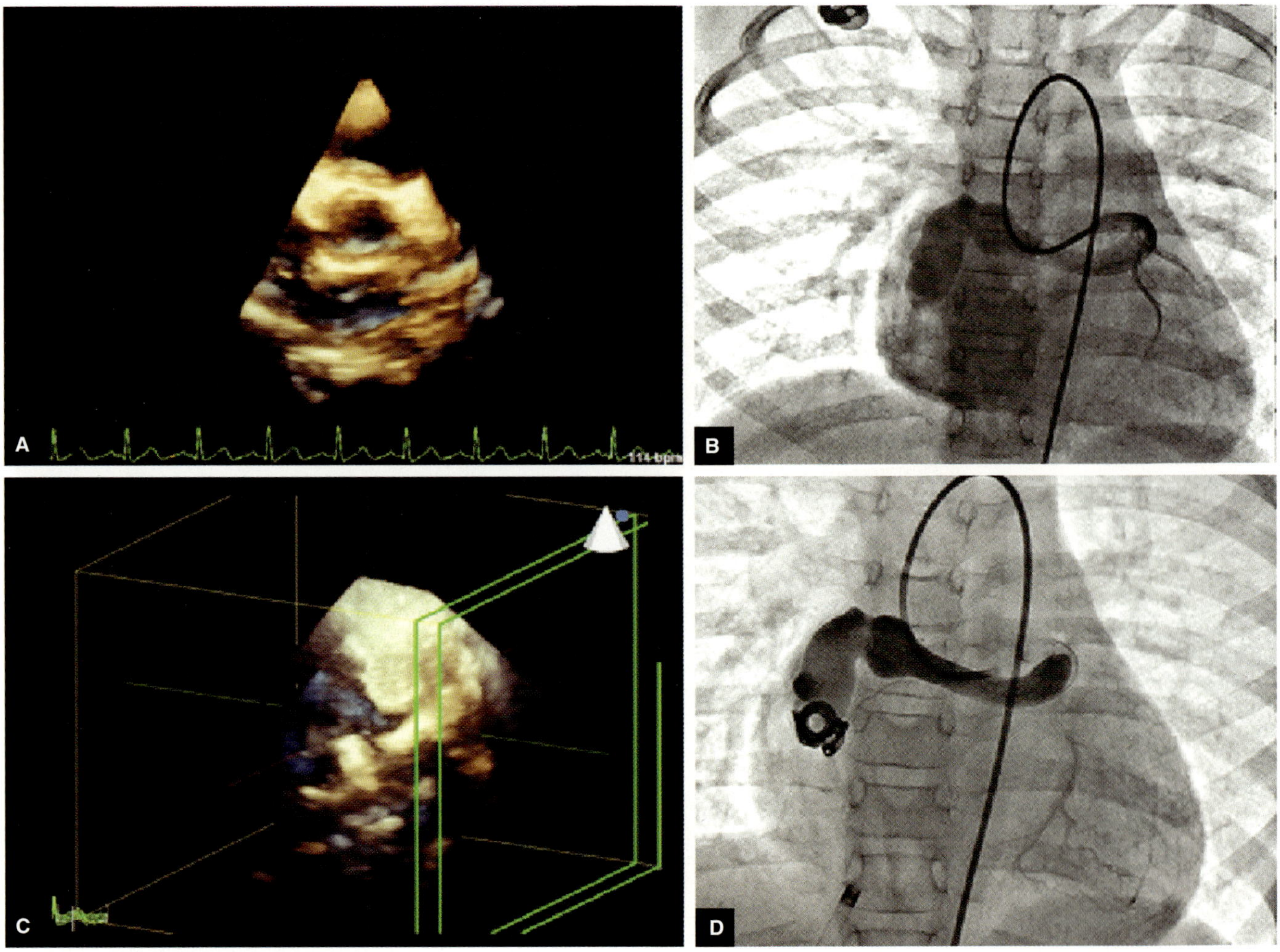

Figure 6: A case of Coronary AV Fistula. (A) Showing the origin of the fistulous track from the left coronary sinus. (B) Showing the same draining into the RA by fluoroscopy. (C) Showing the coils deployed in the fistulous track at its exit point by 3D echo and (D) Showing the same by fluoroscopy

Transthoracic echocardiography (TTE) is the conventional approach for intraprocedural echocardiographic monitoring of transcoronary ablation of septal hypertrophy for HOCM. Some laboratories prefer TEE because it provides more precise imaging of the subaortic anatomy of the left ventricle than TTE.

If TTE is used, apical 4-chamber and 3-chamber (long-axis) views should be used. These views may be supplemented with parasternal long-axis and short-axis views. If TEE is used, the apical 4-chamber view (at 0°) and the longitudinal view (usually 120–130°) should be used. These views may be supplemented by the transgastric short-axis view to help ensure that no erroneous perfusion of the papillary muscles occurs. The deep transgastric view, which resembles an apical 4-chamber transthoracic view, is useful for measuring the intracavitary gradient with TEE.

ECHOCARDIOGRAPHY GUIDED PERICARDIOCENTESIS

Pericardiocentesis is a common day to day procedure that has long relied upon electrocardiographic needle monitoring. However, the complications of such a procedure is damage to the myocardium, lung, coronary arteries and the liver (Figure 7). The incidence of major complications have been dramatically reduced by performance under echocardiographic guidance, ~1.2% in mayo clinic series.[17] The safety and efficacy of echocardiography-guided pericardiocentesis had been shown

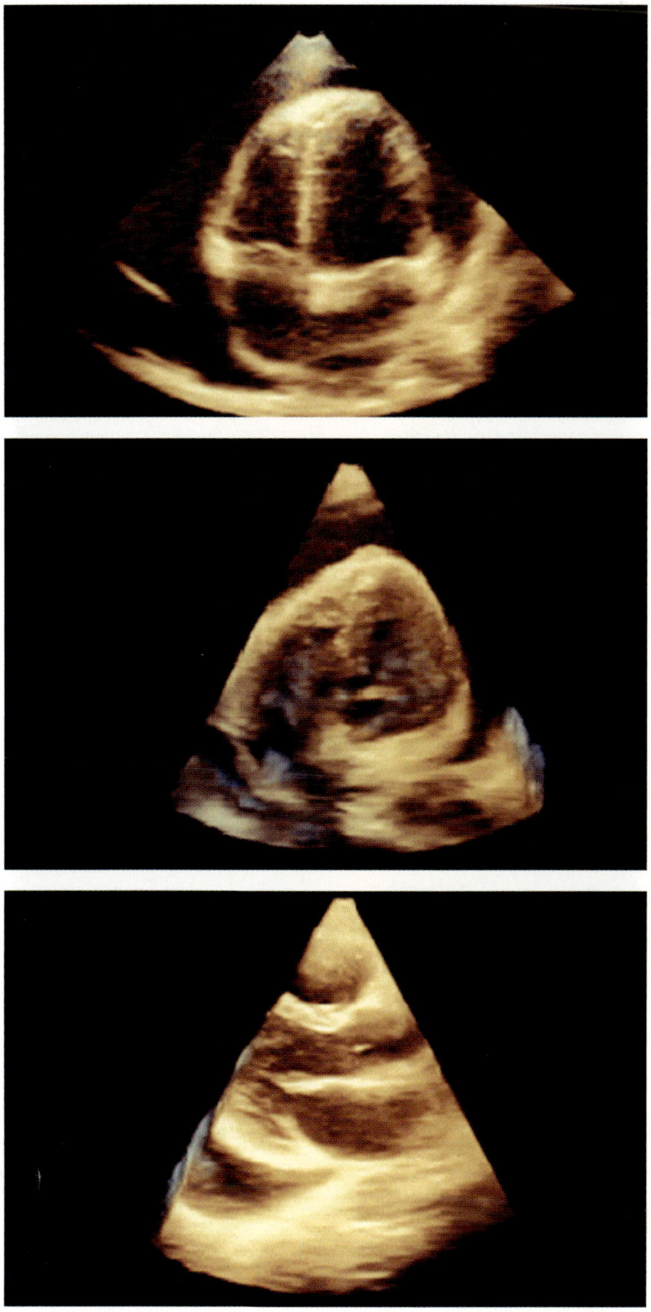

Figure 7: Pericardial effusion demonstrated by 3D

in various subgroups, including pediatric patients, patients who were hemodynamically very unstable after cardiac perforation secondary to invasive percutaneous procedures, postoperative patients, and patients with malignancies or connective tissue diseases.

The subcostal route is routinely selected in most of the centers and it involves a longer path to reach the fluid, passes anterior to the liver capsule, and is directed toward the right chambers of the heart. The position of a catheter introduced into the pericardial space can be confirmed by the injection of agitated saline. The appearance of contrast in the pericardial sac confirms its position. The indwelling catheter is removed once the drainage has decreased (<25 mL in 24 hours) and follow-up echocardiography reveals no significant residual effusion.

ADVANTAGES OF 3D TEE IN BIOPSY PROCEDURES

3D imaging, offers the potential to contribute significantly to interventional procedures. For example, myocardial biopsy has been performed with 3D imaging as a guide for bioptome position (as opposed to the standard approach with fluoroscopy). In one study of 63 routine right ventricular biopsy procedures in cardiac allograft recipients, 3D imaging was deemed feasible, and improved localization of the bioptome was observed, with the potential to improve cardiac biopsy efficacy and safety.[16]

ADVANTAGES OF 3D TEE FOR MITRAL VALVE REPAIR

Mitral valve anatomy may be better studied with 3D imaging than with 2D imaging, and therefore, 3D imaging can play a significant role in the planning of surgical or percutaneous approaches to mitral valve repair.[17] Human studies with intraoperative 3D TEE have shown excellent correlation with surgical findings (94% [34 of 36 patients]) in the correct identification of scallop or segment prolapse. It is expected that 3D echocardiography will play a role in the planning of percutaneous mitral repair of MR. Real-time 3D echocardiography has also been successfully used to guide the surgical approach to myectomy and mitral valve repair in 10 patients in whom a "surgeon's view" by 3D echocardiography allowed refinement of the planned surgical approach.

FUTURE PERSPECTIVES

INTRACARDIAC ECHOCARDIOGRAPHY (ICE)

A more recent application of cardiac ultrasound, ICE has also demonstrated great potential for monitoring and guiding interventions. Experimental and clinical studies have demonstrated the utility of ICE in monitoring left ventricular and right ventricular function, delineating anatomy, guiding transseptal punctures and therapy, and biopsy of cardiac masses.

REFERENCES

1. ASE recommendations for clinical practice, Echocardiography guided interventions; Frank E silvestry; 2009.
2. Hurrell DG, Nishimura RA, Symanski JD, et al. Echocardiography in the invasive laboratory: utility of two-dimensional echocardiography in performing transseptal catheterization. Mayo Clin Proc 1998;73:126-31.
3. Kronzon I, Glassman E, Cohen M, et al. Use of two-dimensional echocardiography during transseptal cardiac catheterization. J Am Coll Cardiol 1984;4:425-8.
4. Pandian NG, Isner JM, Hougen TJ, et al. Percutaneous balloon valvuloplasty of mitral stenosis aided by cardiac ultrasound. Am J Cardiol 1987;59:380-1.
5. Goldstein SA, Campbell AN. Mitral stenosis: evaluation and guidance of valvuloplasty by transesophageal echocardiography. Cardiol Clin 1993;11:409-25.
6. Waksmonski CA, McKay RG. Echocardiographic diagnosis of valve disruption following percutaneous balloon valvuloplasty. Echocardiography 1989;6:277-81.
7. Applebaum RM, Kasliwal RR, Kanojia A, et al. Utility of three-dimensional echocardiography during balloon mitral valvuloplasty. J Am Coll Cardiol 1998;32:1405-9.
8. Park SH, Kim MA, Hyon MS. The advantages of on-line transesophageal echocardiography guide during percutaneous balloon mitral valvuloplasty. J Am Soc Echocardiogr 2000;13:26-34.
9. 3D TEE for Evaluation of Commissural Opening Before and During Percutaneous Mitral Commissurotomy, Edward A Gill, J Am Coll Cardiol Img 2009;2:1034-5.
10. Messika-Zeitoun D, Blanc J, Iung B, et al. Impact of degree of commissural opening after percutaneous mitral commissurotomy on long-term outcome. J Am Coll Cardiol Img 2009;2:1-7.
11. Cooke JC. Echocardiologists' role in the deployment of the Amplatzer atrial septal occluder device in adults. J Am Soc Echocardiogr 2001;14:588-94.
12. Maeno Y, Benson L, Boutin C. Impact of dynamic 3D transesophageal echocardiography in the assessment of atrial septal defects and occlusion by the double-umbrella device (CardioSEAL). Cardiol Young 1998;8:368-78.
13. Sinha A, Nanda NC, Misra V, et al. Live three-dimensional transthoracic echocardiographic assessment of transcatheter closure of atrial septal defect and patent foramen ovale. Echocardiography 2004;21:749-53.
14. Sigwart U. Non-surgical myocardial reduction for hypertrophic obstructive cardiomyopathy. Lancet 1995;346:211-4.
15. McCreery CJ, McCulloch M, Ahmad M, et al. Real-time 3-dimensional echocardiography imaging for right ventricular endomyocardial biopsy: a comparison with fluoroscopy. J Am Soc Echocardiogr 2001;14:927-33.
16. Ahmed S, Nanda NC, Miller AP, et al. Usefulness of transesophageal three-dimensional echocardiography in the identification of individual segment/scallop prolapse of the mitral valve. Echocardiography 2003;20:203-9.
17. Tsang T, Enriquez-Sarano M, Freeman W, et al. Consecutive 1127 therapeutic echocardiographically guided pericardio-centeses: clinical profile, practice patterns, and outcomes spanning 21 years. Mayo Clin Proc 2002;77:429-36.

CHAPTER 10

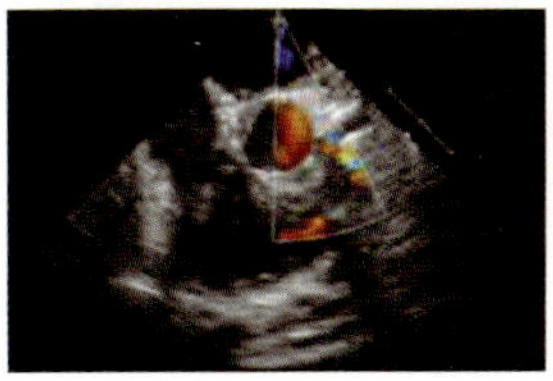

Anomalous Origin of Left Coronary Artery from Pulmonary Artery

V Amuthan, RA Janarthanan, S Balasubramanian, P Ashok Kumar

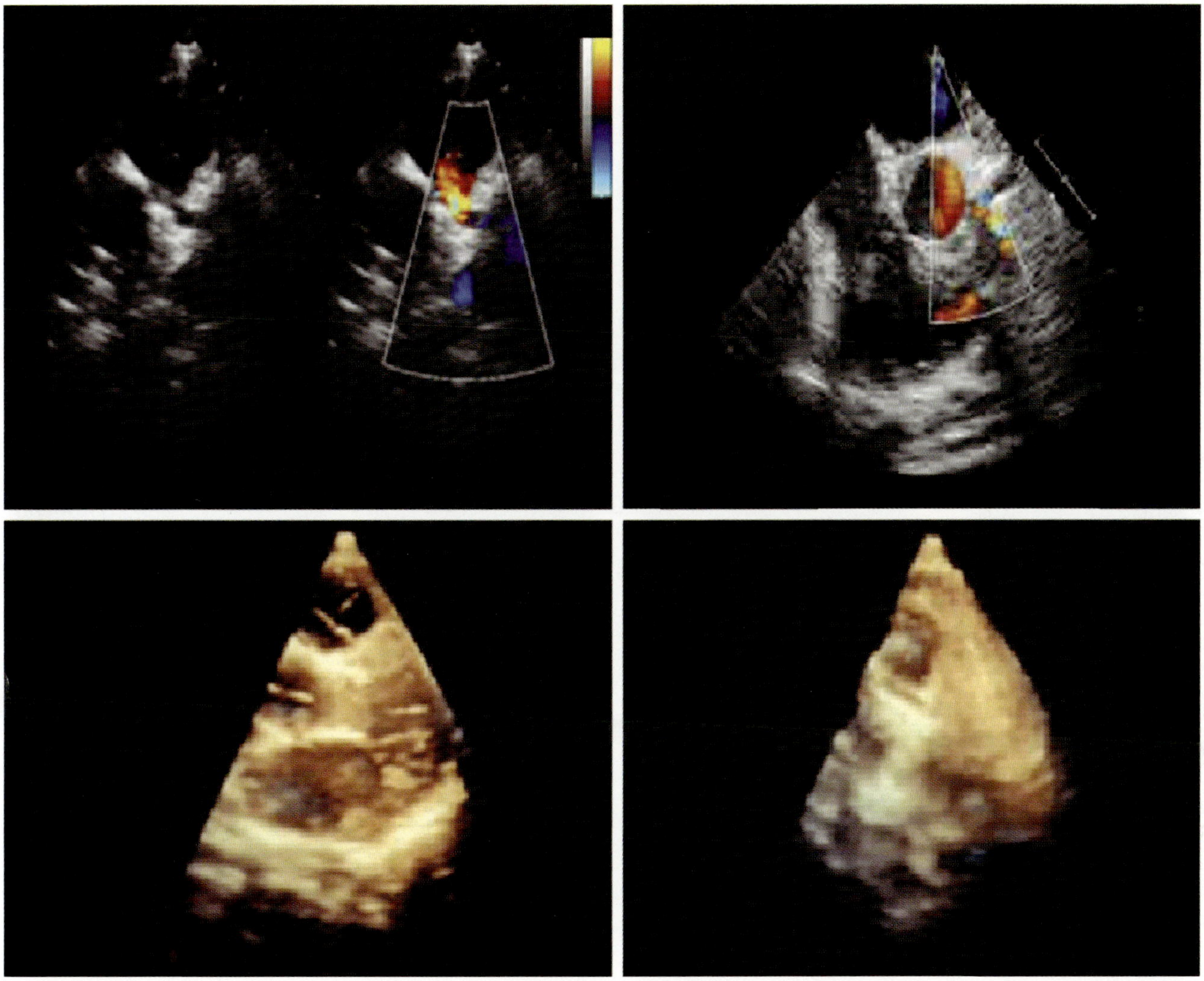

Figure 1: **Top left :** 2D Echo short axis view showing anomalous left coronary artery arising from main pulmonary artery with left to right shunt
Top Right : Trans Esophageal Echocardiography again showing the MPA below and the anomalous LCA with left to right shunt
Bottom Right and left : 3D Echo showing the anomalous left coronary artery arising from main pulmonary artery

INTRODUCTION

Anomalous origin of left coronary artery from pulmonary artery (ALCAPA) also known as Bland White Garland Syndrome is a rare congenital heart disease with an incidence of about 1 in 300,000 live births.[1,6] The presentation is during infancy in 85% of the patients. Early childhood mortality occurs due to heart failure and SCD. Fifteen percent of the cases present late and reach 3rd to 4th decade.[1] If collateral circulation between right and left coronary systems ensues, ALCAPA patients may reach adulthood. However, coronary flow directs preferentially into the lower pressure PA, away from the left ventricle (LV) creating "coronary steal", and left-to-right shunt.[4,7] Angiography was the main modality for diagnosis until the advent of echocardiography which has almost replaced angiography. The advent of 3D echocardiography has thrown more light into the noninvasive diagnosis of ALCAPA.

CASE REPORT

7 year old school boy presented with H/O chest discomfort and shortness of breath of 6 months duration. He was apparently normal prior to that. He was born of a full term normal delivery and development was normal with no history of cyanosis, feeding difficulties or cyanotic spells. On examination, patient was comfortable at rest. He was not anemic and there was no clubbing or cyanosis. Cardiovascular examination revealed normal pulses and Jugular venous pulse and pressure. The precordium was quite and the apical impulse was in normal location. Auscultation revealed a continuous murmur in right 2nd, 3rd, left 3rd intercostal space. Chest X-ray was normal.

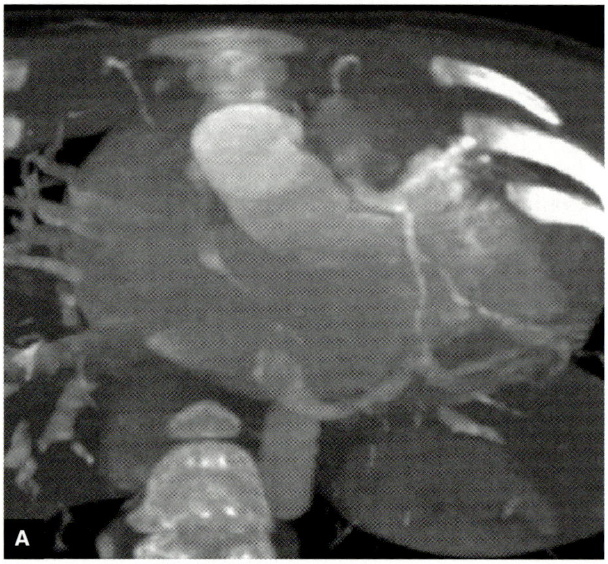

Figure 2A: CT angiogram showing the origin of LCA from the pulmonary artery

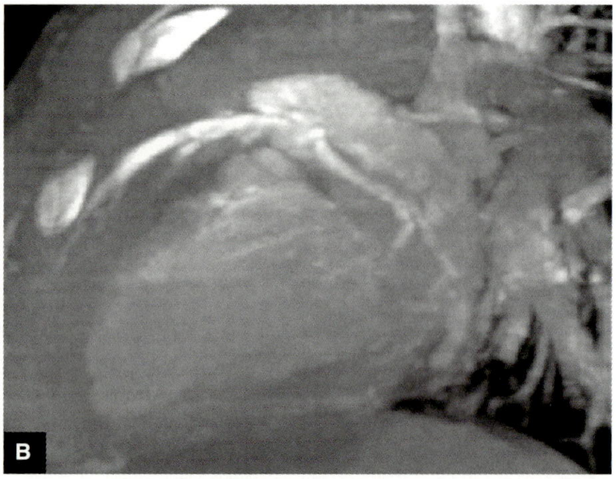

Figure 2B: CT Angiogram showing the dilated LCA arising from the pulmonary artery

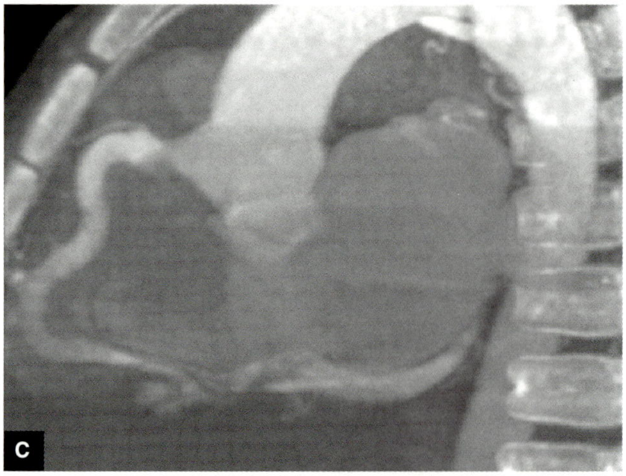

Figure 2C: CT Angiogram showing the origin of dilated RCA from the right aortic sinus

DISCUSSION

The physiology of ALCAPA is described under the following nonchronological phases:[3,8,9]

i. The phase of high pulmonary vascular resistance (PVR) and pulmonary artery pressure (PAP) as is seen in the newborn period. There are no symptoms or signs of ischemia.
ii. A transition phase during which the PVR and PAP fall, flow becomes retrograde and unless collaterals develop there are signs of ischemia.

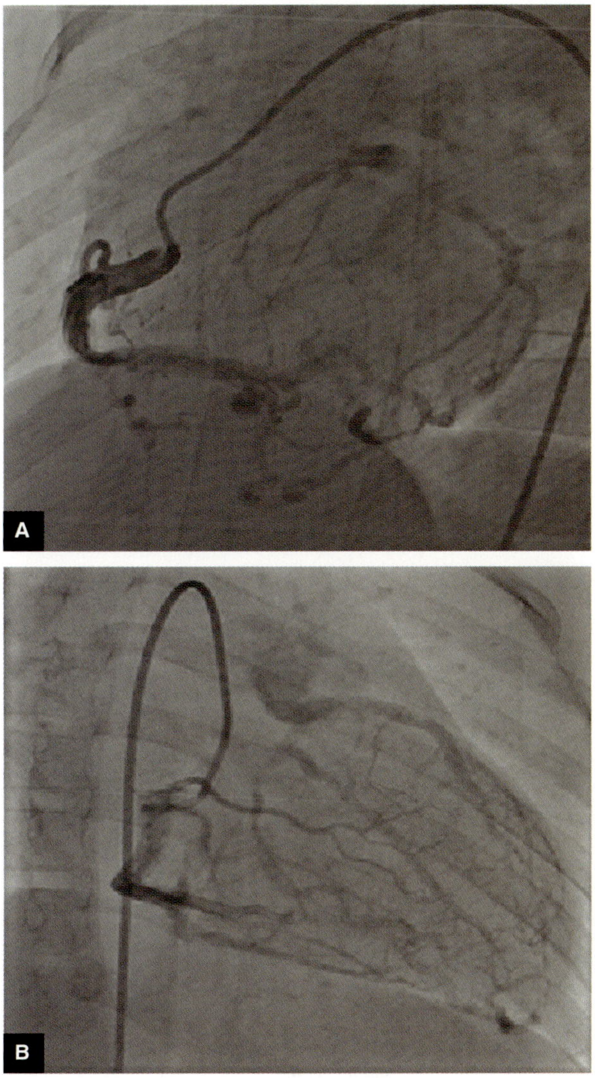

Figures 3A and B: Coronary angiogram in LAO and RAO projection showing the origin of RCA from the right coronary sinus and filling of the LCA from the RCA during the Levo phase

iii. Adult phase during which adequate collaterals develop and again there are no signs of ischemia.

iv. The LCA is no longer a feeding vessel and just acts as a conduit. There is coronary steal; and hence signs of ischemia.

Echocardiography has replaced angiography as a tool for the diagnosis of ALCAPA. 2D echo shows the anomalous origin of left coronary artery from the pulmonary trunk.[2,5] However the diagnosis rests on the demonstration of color flow reversal in the coronary arteries. The criteria are a dilated right coronary system with flow reversal in at least two of the three left coronary segments. There is a flow reversal into the pulmonary trunk with the turbulence along the medial wall as against the lateral wall in a patent ductus. The location of left coronary segments and demonstration of flow reversal is however difficult (Figure 1).

Transesophageal echocardiography (TEE), mid-esophageal aortic valve long axis view can demonstrate the large orifice of the right coronary artery with laminar diastolic antegrade flow by color Doppler mapping.[2,5]

3D echo can clearly delineate the coronary system than the conventional 2D echocardiography and make the diagnosis of ALCAPA simpler (Figure 1 Lower panels).

Other valuable noninvasive technique is coronary CT angiogram. We can demonstrate the origin of RCA alone from the right coronary sinus whereas the left coronary sinus is devoid of any coronary origin. Instead the left coronary artery is seen to originate from the pulmonary artery (Figures 2. A, B & C).

Cardiac catheterization also reveals the absence of the LMCA in the left sinus of valsalva. Contrast dye injected into the right coronary artery (RCA) fills the main branches of the LMCA with anomalous drainage through the LMCA into the PA (Figure 3). Management of ALCAPA has evolved dramatically over the years. Management is surgical. Initial days saw bypass grafting procedures using the Subclavian artery. Now, most preferred treatment is the reimplantation of the left coronary artery into the aortic sinus. Rarely, aortopulmonary window with a tunnel to divert the blood into the left coronary artery is used.

REFERENCES

1. Keith JD. Anomalous origin of left coronary from pulmonary artery. Br Heart J 1959;21:149.
2. Houston AB, Pollock JCS, Doig WB, et al. ALCAPA elucidation with colour Doppler flow mapping Br H J. 1990; 63:50.
3. Huritz RA, Caldwell RL Clinical and hemodynamic course of infants and children with ALCAPA. Am H J. 1989;118:1176.
4. Askenazi J, Nadas AS. Report of 15 cases of ALCAPA, circulation 1975;51:976.
5. International Anesthesia research society. 2007;6:104.
6. Coronary anomalies. Circulation 2002;105:2449-54.
7. ACC/AHA 2008 Guidelines for the Management of Adults with Congenital Heart Disease. Circulation 2008;118;e714-e833.
8. The science and practice of pediatric cardiology by Garzon ed.
9. Recognition of congenital heart disease in adults. Joseph K perlof 5 ed.

CHAPTER 11

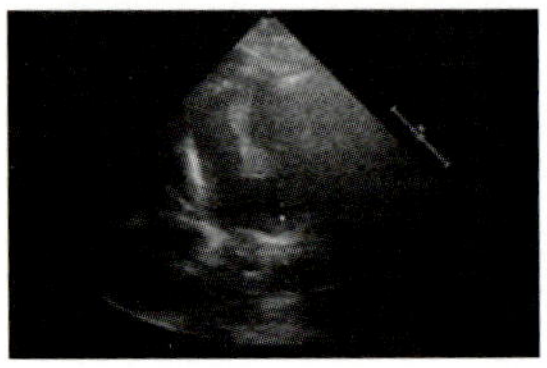

Advantages of 3D Echo over 2D Echo in Assessment of LV Clot in Patients with Myocardial Infarction

C Balachandran, V Amuthan, RA Janarthanan, S Balasubramanian
S Naina Mohamed, N Ganesan, P Ashok Kumar, SR Veeramani, R Aravazhi

ABSTRACT

Left ventricular thrombus is a well recognized complication of acute myocardial infarction. The prevention recognition and appropriate treatment of this condition remain important because of the potential risk of systemic embolisation. Transthoracic echocardiography (TTE) remains the most common imaging modality to make a diagnosis of left ventricular thrombus. Advantages of TTE include convenience, portability, wide availability, relatively low cost compared to other imaging modalities, and the ability to provide important ancillary information on cardiac structure and function. The aim of the study was to find out the advantage of 3D echo over 2D echo in assessing LV clot in patients with myocardial infarction. There were ninety four patients admitted as myocardial infarction between January 2009 to July 2009. Among them eighty-two were males and twelve were females. All patients were subjected to both 2D echo and 3D echo between 2 days and 5 days after myocardial infarction. The LV dimensions, LV volumes, mitral regurgitation, ventricular septal rupture, LV clot were the variables, which were studied.

INTRODUCTION

Left ventricular thrombus (LVT) is a well-recognized complication of acute myocardial infarction (AMI) due to severely impaired LV systolic function.[1-3] While the current use of antiplatelet and anticoagulant medications in these patient populations may have reduced the prevalence of LV thrombi, the prevention, recognition, and appropriate treatment of this condition remain important because of the potential risk of systemic embolization.

Left ventricular thrombus formation is a frequent complication observed in patients following an AMI and in those with systolic heart failure due to Dilated Cardiomyopathy.[5,6] Previously, the incidence of LVT was reported to be as high as 30 to 40% in patients with an anterior AMI. For patients with a nonanterior AMI, the risk of LVT was lower (<5%).[4] Although controversial, in the contemporary era of routine early revascularization and more aggressive anticoagulation, the incidence of LVT complicating an anterior AMI is likely reduced and is currently estimated at 5 to 15%.[2,3] The prevention, diagnosis, and appropriate treatment of LVT are important because of the increased risk of systemic embolization, particularly, cardio embolic stroke.[9-12] Although two-dimensional transthoracic echocardiography is the standard in diagnosis of LV thrombus, Real time 3-dimensional echocardiography adds one more dimension and has been described to be more sensitive.[13] Newer modalities for diagnosis of left ventricular thrombus such as platelets labeled with indium 111, contrast enhanced CT imaging, magnetic resonance imaging radionuclide angiography are now available.[14-19] Nevertheless because of its wide availability, inexpensiveness, and lack of radiation exposure echocardiography remains the modality of choice for diagnosing left ventricular thrombus.

MATERIALS AND METHODS

The study population consisted of ninety-four patients with acute ST elevation myocardial infarction admitted in the intensive care coronary care unit in government Rajaji hospital between January 2009 to July 2009. Patients were treated with thrombolytic agents if there were no contraindications. Between two and five days they were subjected to both 2D echo and 3D echo. The following groups of patients were excluded from the study. Post infarction angina, presence of LBBB, and unstable angina. Echocardiography was done using Phillips IE 33 machine having 2D and 3D echo facility.

All eligible patients underwent basic investigations and subjected to echocardiography. Since the propensity for thrombi is to form at the apex of the LV, the best imaging plane to visualize left ventricular thrombus are the apical views where the transducer is closest to the region of interest. This also eliminates certain normal anatomic structures (papillary muscles, falsetendons, trabeculations) and technical artifacts (reverberations and near field artifacts) that will result in false positive diagnosis of left ventricular thrombus. So we used higher frequency transducers that has shown to overcome some of these limitations due to higher spatial resolution and reduced artifacts (Figure 1). The parameters assessed in 2D echo were the assessment of regional wall motion abnormality, left ventricular end diastolic volume and end systolic volumes, wall thickness during diastole and systole, presence of mitral regurgitation, presence of ventricular septal rupture, presence of spontaneous echo contrast, apical rotating flow, vortex ring formation, and left ventricular clot.

Finally by using newer real-time 3D echocardiographic techniques we were able to demonstrate better characterization and delineation of the extent of LVT.[13] Three-dimensional echocardiography has been developed in several steps since the initial development of 3D echocardiography. Transthoracic data acquisition with the rotation procedure or the free hand technique was realized. The limited image realization of these procedures has been clearly improved by recent developments. The limited image resolution of these procedures have been clearly improved by recent developments. The decisive disadvantage of these procedures however remains that the data acquisition and presentation are not done in real time. The introduction of the phased real-time volumetric imaging enabled real-time acquisition of 3D echocardiographic data sets. A breakthrough in the area of transthoracic real time 3D echocardiography was received with so called live 3D technique. Using live 3D TTE, the thrombus was easily viewed end-on and from the sides. In addition, by cropping the 3D images sequentially in transverse (horizontal or short axis), longitudinal (vertical or long axis), frontal, and oblique planes, the degree and extent of lysis within the thrombus, which represents an integral part of the clot resolution process, was assessed.

By cropping of a single 3D TTE apical dataset we were able to provide comprehensive assessment of the LV in a timely manner even without breath holding in a not fully cooperative patient.

We identified the exact point of attachment of the thrombus to the left ventricular wall.

Focal echo lucent areas within thrombi were analyzed indicative of the presence and extent of clot lysis, which may have potential therapeutic and prognostic implications. Accurate assessment of thrombus mobility was assessed which has prognostic indications. The number of left ventricular thrombus was best assessed by useing three dimensional Echocardiography.

Statistical analysis and results in our study of 94 patients. 48 patients had anterior wall myocardial infarction and 46 patients had inferior wall myocardial infarction. The mean LVEF in patients without a LVCLOT was 46.6±10.48 the mean LVEF in patients with LVCLOT 37.4±9.26 by 3D echo method. By the 2D echo method the values were

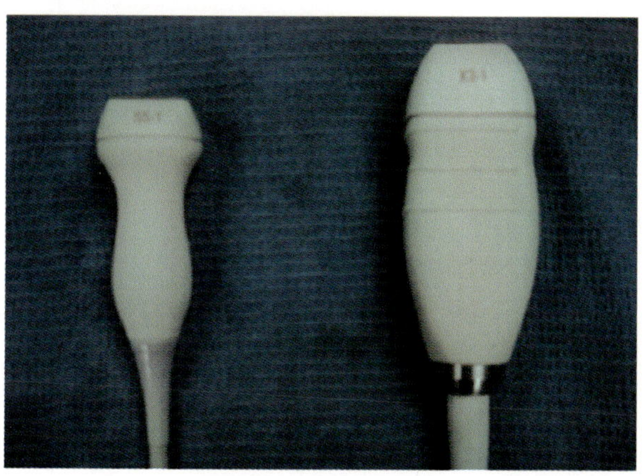

Figure 1: 2D and 3D probes used in this study

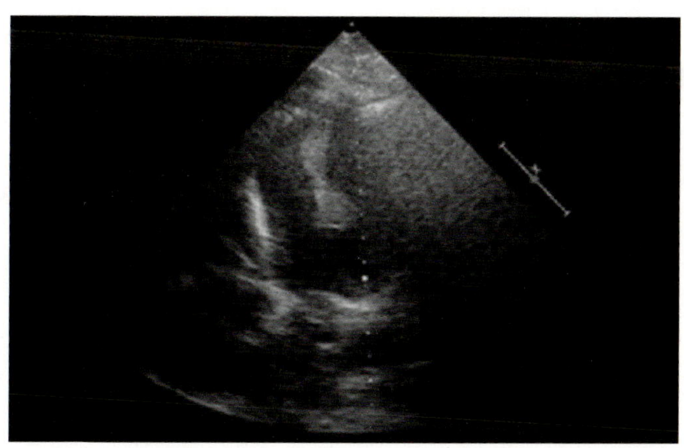

Figure 2: LV clot demonstration by 2D echo

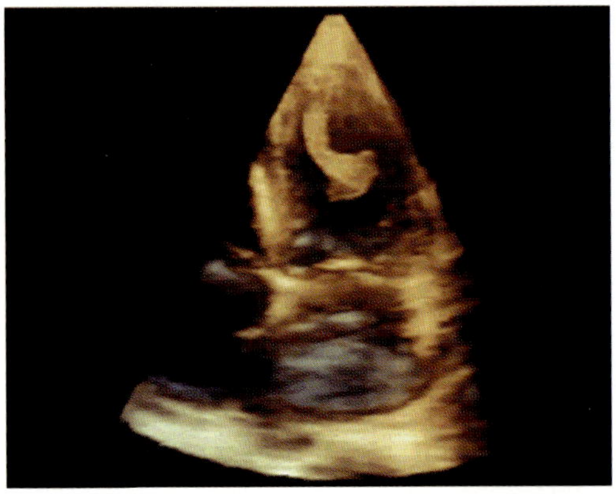

Figure 3: LV clot demonstration by 3D echo

49±12.6 in patients without a LVCLOT and 45.28±1.28 in patients with a LVCLOT. Mitral Regurgitation was seen in 51.8% by 3D echo and 38% by 2D echo. Ventricular Septal Rupture was seen in 10% of cases. LV CLOT was seen in 22 patients by 3D echo method and sensitivity is 100%. By 2D echo only 18 patients had LV CLOT and sensitivity is 60%. Two patients had more than one LV CLOT that is visualized only in 3D echo (Table 1). Left ventricular thrombus is more common in patients presenting with acute anterior wall myocardial infarction rather than patients presenting with inferior wall myocardial infarction. Among forty-eight patients with anterior wall myocardial infarction seventeen patients had left ventricular thrombus. Among forty-six patients with inferior wall myocardial infarction left ventricular thrombus was seen in only five patients. The sensitivity of detecting left ventricular thrombus by three-dimensional echocardiography is comparatively more than that of two-dimensional echocardiography (Figures 2 and 3).

DISCUSSION

Left ventricular thrombus (LVT) formation is a frequent complication observed in patients following an AMI and in those with systolic CHF. Previously, the incidence of LVT was reported to be as high as 30 to 40% in patients with an anterior AMI. For patients with a nonanterior AMI, the risk of LVT was lower (<5%).[4] Although controversial, in the contemporary era of routine early revascularization and more aggressive anticoagulation, the incidence of LVT complicating an anterior AMI is likely reduced and is currently estimated at 5 to 15% (Table 2).[2-4] The prevention, diagnosis, and appropriate treatment of LVT are important because of the increased risk of systemic embolization, particularly, cardio embolic stroke. Transthoracic echocardiography (TTE) remains the most common imaging modality to make a diagnosis of LVT. Advantages of TTE include convenience, portability, wide availability, relatively low cost compared to other imaging modalities, and the ability to provide important ancillary information on cardiac structure and function. When images are technically adequate, TTE has a

TABLE 1 Echocardiographic Data

	AWMI	*IWMI*	*Total*	*Mean LVEF (No clot)*	*Mean LVEF (With clot)*	*MR*	*VSR*	*Single LV clot*	*More than one clot*	*Sensitivity*	
										Single LV clot	*> 1 LV clot*
3D echo	48	46	94	46.6 ± 10.48	37.4 ± 9.26	51.8%	10%	22	2	100%	100%
2D echo	48	46	94	49 ± 12.6	45.28 ± 1.28	38%	10%	18	0	60%	

TABLE 2 LV clot in thrombolysed vs non thrombolysed patients

	AWMI				*IWMI*			
	Thrombolysed		*Not Thrombolysed*		*Thrombolysed*		*Not Thrombolysed*	
	Clot	*No clot*	*Clot*	*No clot*	*Clot*	*No clot*	*Clot*	*No clot*
3D echo	10 (33%)	20 (67%)	7 (39%)	11 (61%)	3 (10%)	26 (90%)	2 (12%)	15 (88%)
2D echo	7 (26%)	23 (74%)	7 (39%)	11 (61%)	2 (7%)	27 (93%)	2 (12%)	15 (88%)

sensitivity of 90 to 95% and a specificity of 85 to 90% for detection of LVT in studies where the presence of thrombi was confirmed at surgery or autopsy.[7,8]

ECHOCARDIOGRAPHIC CRITERIA FOR LV THROMBUS

Left ventricular thrombus is a distinct echogenic mass within the LV cavity (may be sessile/layered or protruding/mobile) that is contiguous with, but acoustically distinct from the underlying endocardial surface. It is seen throughout the cardiac cycle and visualized on at least 2 orthogonal views. There is an associated underlying region of severe wall motion abnormality, usually severe hypokinesis, akinesis, dyskinesis, or aneurysmal dilatation.[7-10] The following echocardiographic characteristics of LVT are associated with a higher risk of embolization: Mobility, protrusion and central echo-lucency.[20]

High-risk echocardiographic features for the development of LVT are large infarct size and extent, anterior >>inferior, severe global and regional LV systolic dysfunction, presence of CHF, elevated LV end-systolic volume, LV dilatation, spontaneous echo contrast.

CONCLUSION

Left ventricular thrombus (LVT) remains an important complication in patients with ischemic heart disease after anterior AMI and in those and systolic heart failure. The diagnosis of LVT remains important, since anticoagulation will reduce the risk of systemic embolization and stroke. Despite advances in other imaging modalities, echocardiography remains the most important tool for diagnosis and risk stratification in patients predisposed to developing LVT. While the overall benefit of routine anticoagulation to prevent LVT and stroke remains controversial, in certain select patients who are at a very high-risk for developing LVT and have no contraindications, systemic anticoagulation is generally recommended. The study shows that three-dimensional echocardiography is a useful tool in assessment of left ventricular clot in patients with acute myocardial infarction.

REFERENCES

1. Asinger RW, Mikell FL, Elsperger J, et al. Incidence of left-ventricular thrombosis after acute transmural myocardial infarction. Serial evaluation by two-dimensional echocardiography. N Engl J Med 1981;305:297-302.
2. Kalra A, Jang IK. Prevalence of early left ventricular throm- bus after primary coronary intervention for acute myocardial infarction. J Thromb Thrombolysis 2000;10:133-6.
3. Greaves SC, Zhi G, Lee RT, et al. Incidence and natural his- tory of left ventricular thrombus following anterior wall acute myocardial infarction. Am J Cardiol 1997;80:442-8.
4. Nayak D, Aronow WS, Sukhija R, et al. Comparison of frequency of left ventricular thrombi in patients with anterior wall versus nonanterior wall acute myocardial infarction treated with antithrombotic and antiplatelet therapy with or without coronary revascularization. Am J Cardiol 2004;93:1529-30.
5. Ciaccheri M, Castelli G, Cecchi F, et al. Lack of correlation between intracavitary thrombosis detected by cross sectional echocardiography and systemic emboli in patients with dilated cardiomyopathy. Br Heart J 1989;62:26-9.
6. Gottdiener JS, Gay JA, VanVoorhees L, et al. Frequency and embolic potential of left ventricular thrombus in dilated cardiomyopathy: assessment by 2-dimensional echo-cardiography. Am J Cardiol 1983;52:1281-5.
7. Visser CA, Kan G, David GK, et al. Two-dimensional echocardiography in the diagnosis of left ventricular thrombus. A prospective study of 67 patients with anatomic validation. Chest 1983;83:228-32.
8. Cacciapuoti F, Varrichio M, D'Avino M, et al. Postnecrotic endoventricular thrombosis. Comparative evaluation of the diagnostic reliability of 2-dimensional echocardiography and cineventriculography. G Ital Cardiol 1986;16:344-9.
9. Asinger RW, Mikell FL, Sharma B, et al. Observations on detecting left ventricular thrombus with two-dimensional echocardiography: emphasis on avoidance of false positive diagnoses. Am J Cardiol 1981;47:145-56.
10. Otto CM. The Practice of Clinical Echocardiography. Philadelphia, PA: WB Saunders Company; 2005.
11. Merino A, Hauptman P, Badimon L, et al. Echocardiographic "smoke" is produced by an interaction of erythrocytes and plasma proteins modulated by shear forces. J Am Coll Cardiol 1992;20:1661-8.

12. Ngai T, Atar S, Luo H, et al. The usefulness of second gen- eration ultrasound contrast agents to identify intracardiac thrombus. J Am Coll Cardiol 1999;33:408A.
13. Chamoun AJ, McCulloch M, Xie T, et al. Real-time three-dimensional echocardiography versus two-dimensional echocardiography in the diagnosis of left ventricular apical thrombi: preliminary findings. J Clin Ultrasound 2003;31:412-8.
14. Goldstein JA, Schiller NB, Lipton MJ, et al. Evaluation of left ventricular thrombi by contrast-enhanced computed tomography and two-dimensional echocardiography. Am J Cardiol 1986;57:757-60.
15. Barkhausen J, Hunold P, Eggebrecht H, et al. Detection and characterization of intracardiac thrombi on MR imaging. AJR Am J Roentgenol 2002;179:1539-44.
16. Mollet NR, Dymarkowski S, Volders W, et al. Visualization of ventricular thrombi with contrast-enhanced magnetic resonance imaging in patients with ischemic heart disease. Circulation 2002;106:2873-6.
17. Neskovic AN, Marinkovic J, Bojic M, et al. Predictors of left ventricular thrombus formation and disappearance after anterior wall myocardial infarction. Eur Heart J 1998;19:908-16.
18. Van Dantzig JM, Delemarre BJ, Bot H, et al. Doppler left ventricular flow pattern versus conventional predictors of left ventricular thrombus after acute myocardial infarction. J Am Coll Cardiol 1995;25:1341-6.
19. Vaitkus PT, Barnathan ES. Embolic potential, prevention and management of mural thrombus complicating anterior myocardial infarction: a meta-analysis. J Am Coll Cardiol 1993;22(4):1004-9.
20. Haugland JM, Asinger RW, Mikell FL, et al. Embolic potential of left ventricular thrombi detected by two-dimensional echocardiography. Circulation 1984;70:588-98.

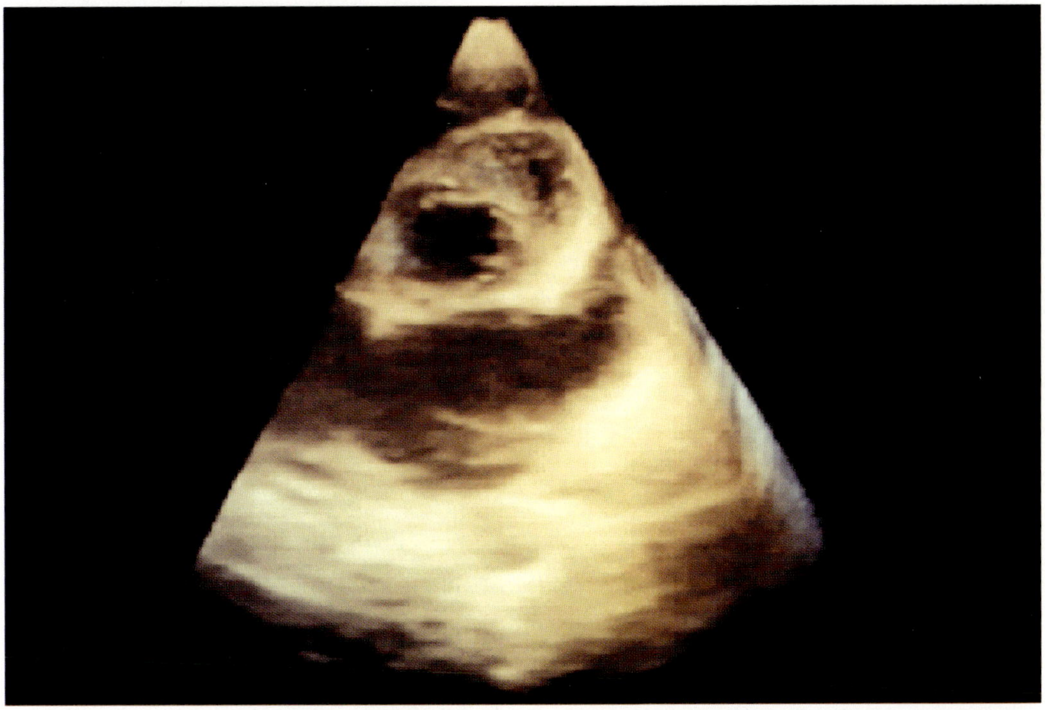

Figure 1: Aortic root abscess

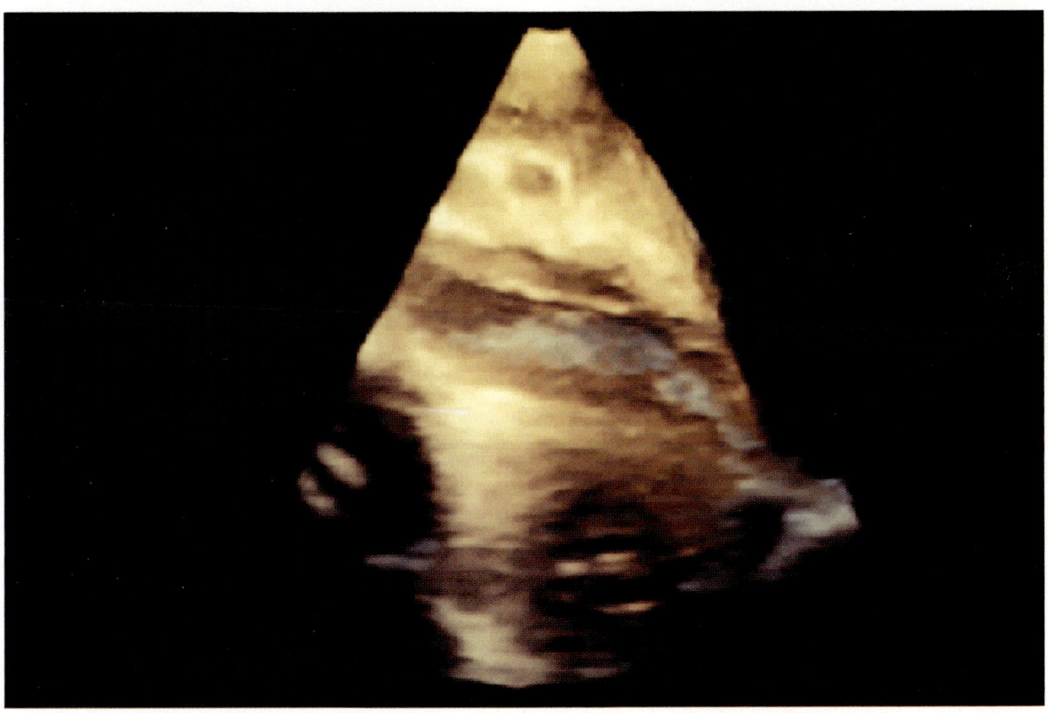

Figure 2: Aortic dissection showing the dissection flap in the abdominal aorta

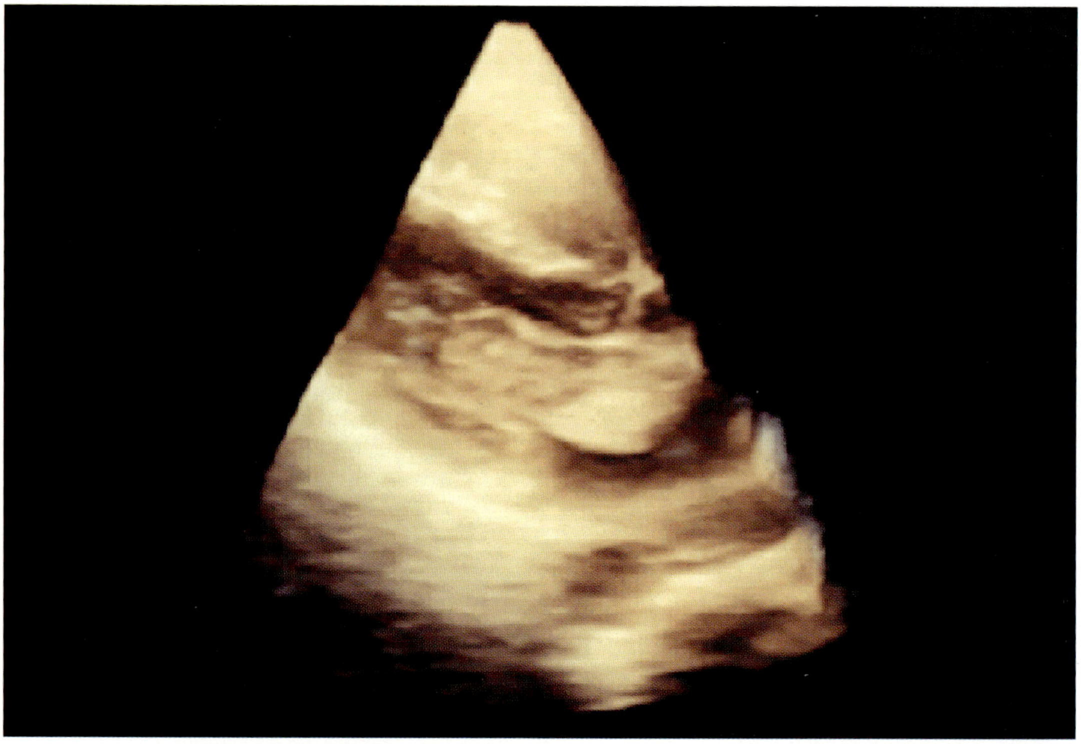

Figure 3: Left atrial myxoma protruding into left ventricle during diastole

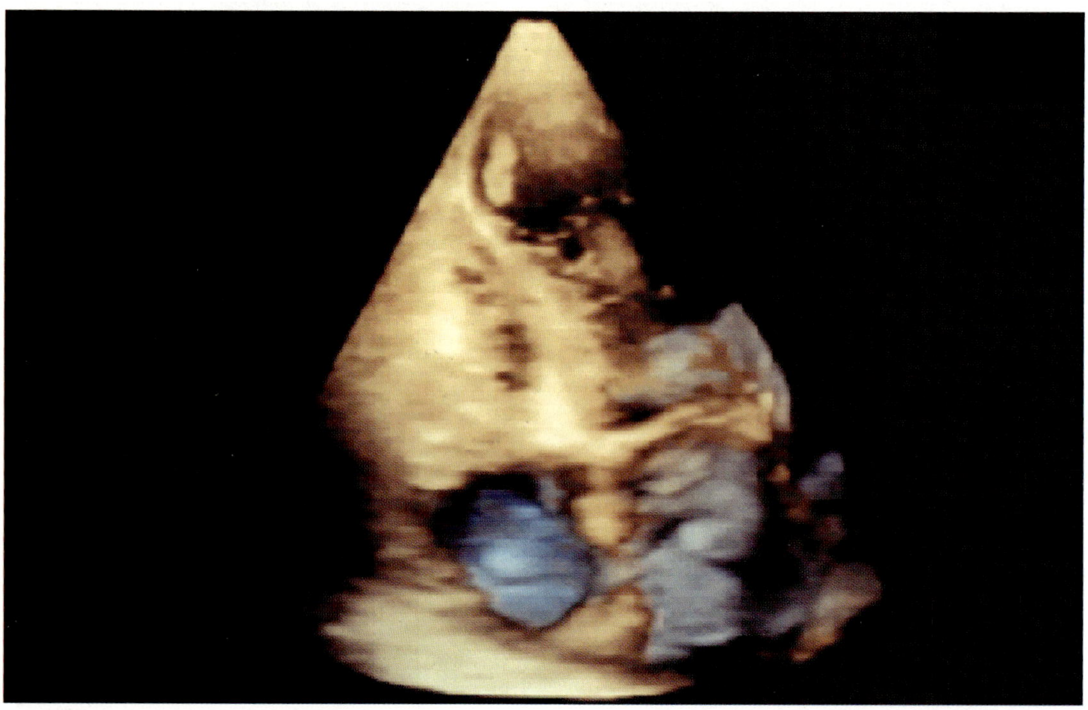

Figure 4: Left ventricular thrombus

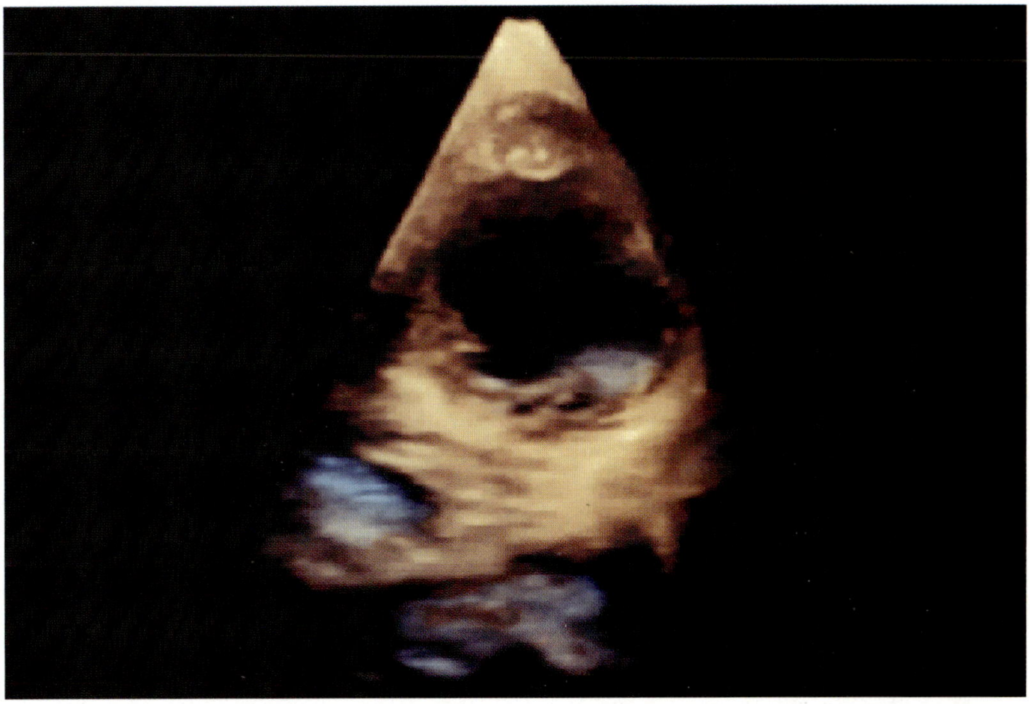

Figure 5: Left ventricular mass

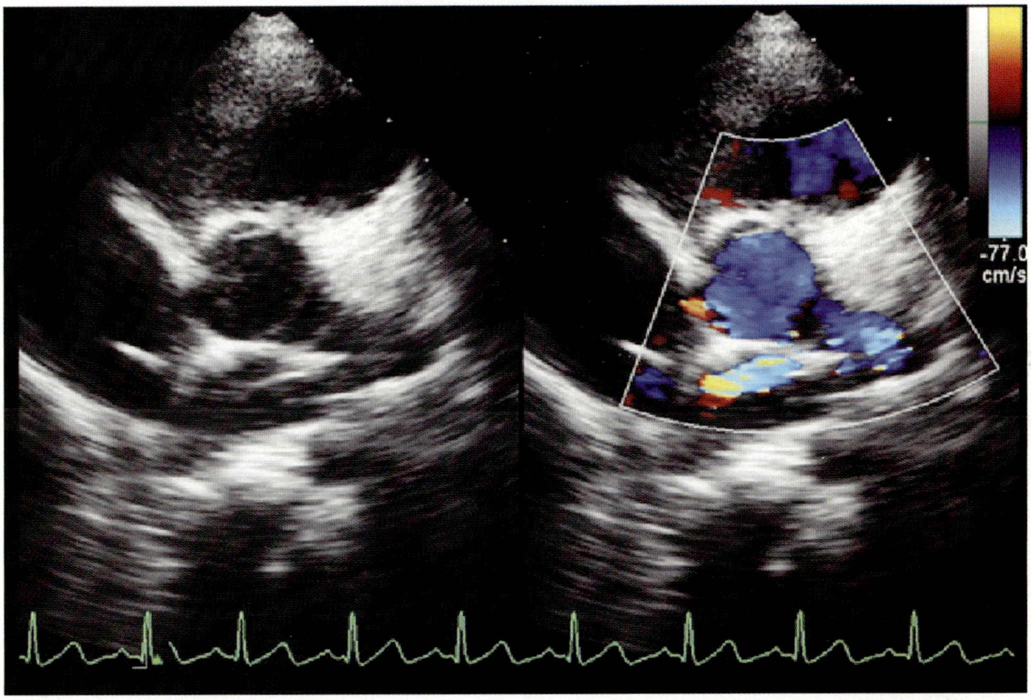

Figure 6: Coronary AV fistula: 2D Color flow image of dilated left coronary artery (LCA) draining into right atrium

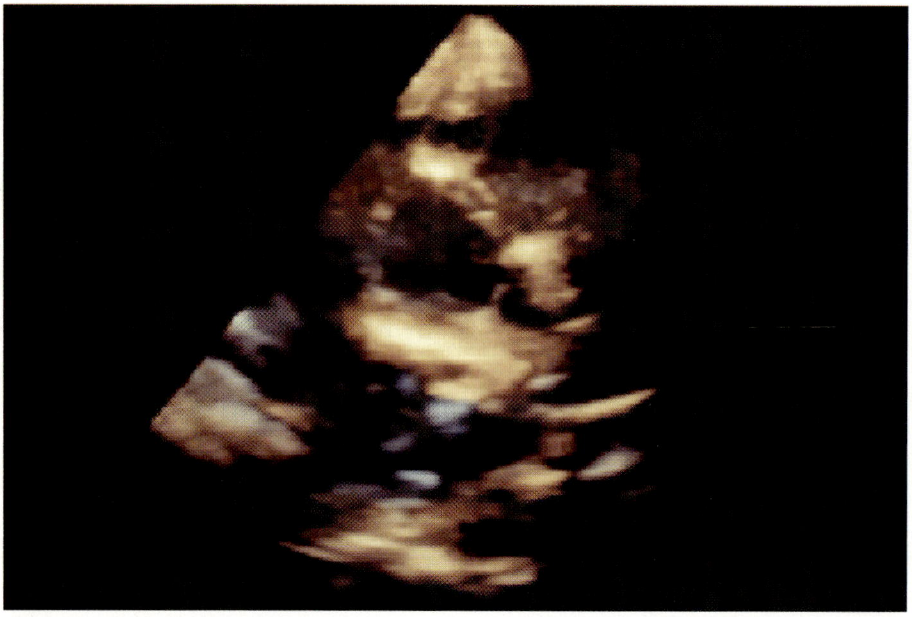

Figure 7: 3D image of the same patient with coronary AV fistula showing dilated left coronary artery

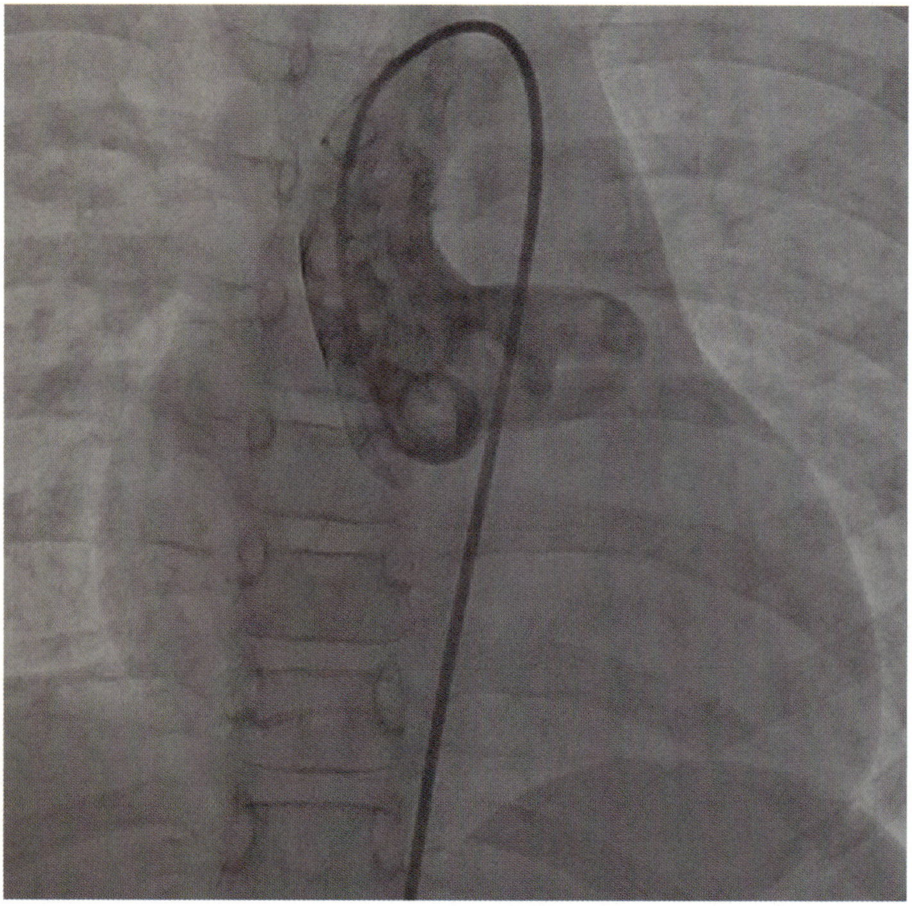

Figure 8: Coronary AV fistula: Aortic root angiogram showing dilated left coronary sinus and left coronary artery

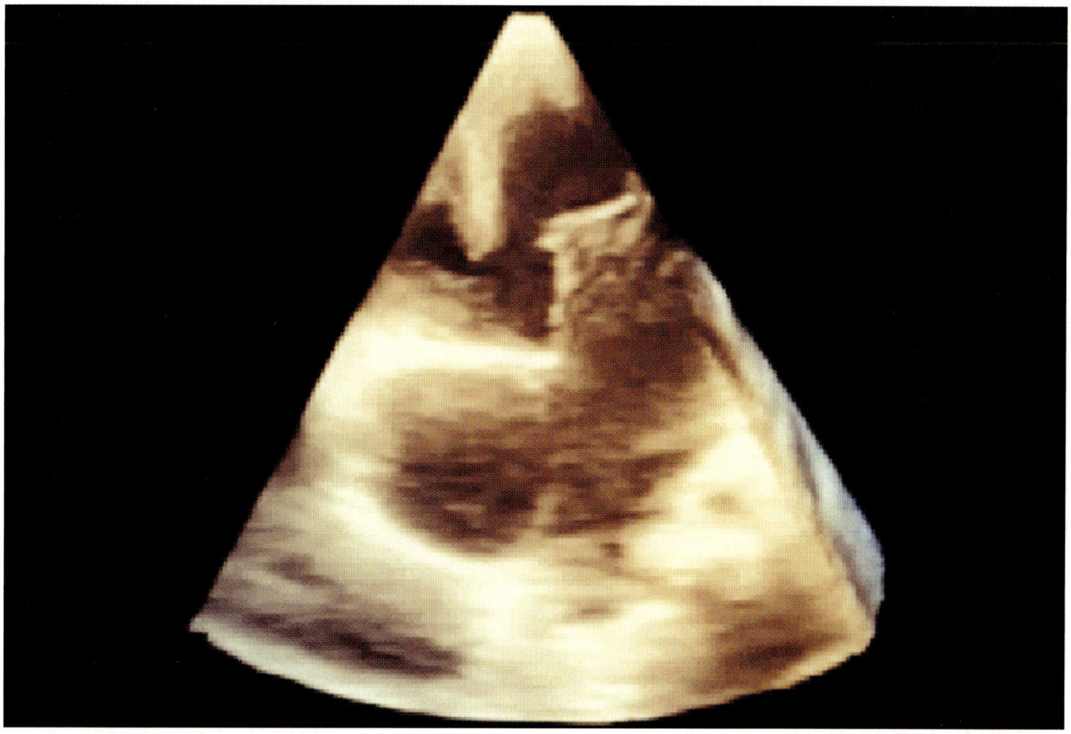

Figure 9: Tricuspid atresia

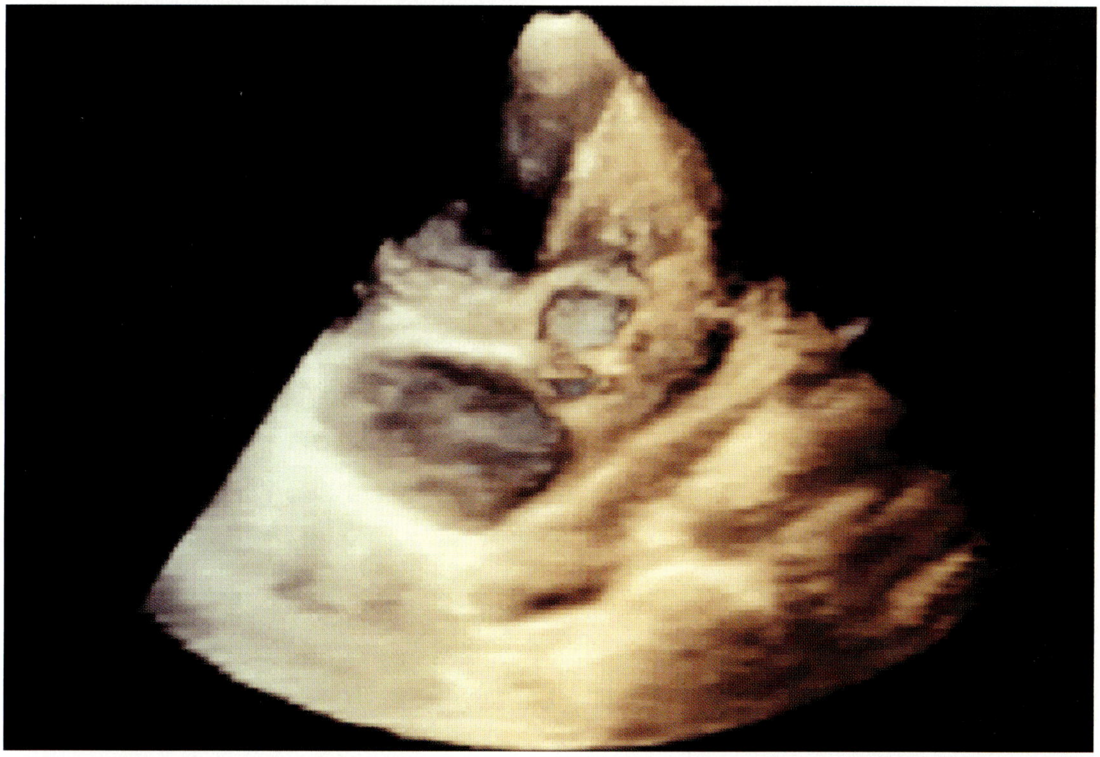

Figure 10: A case of TAPVC showing vertical vein

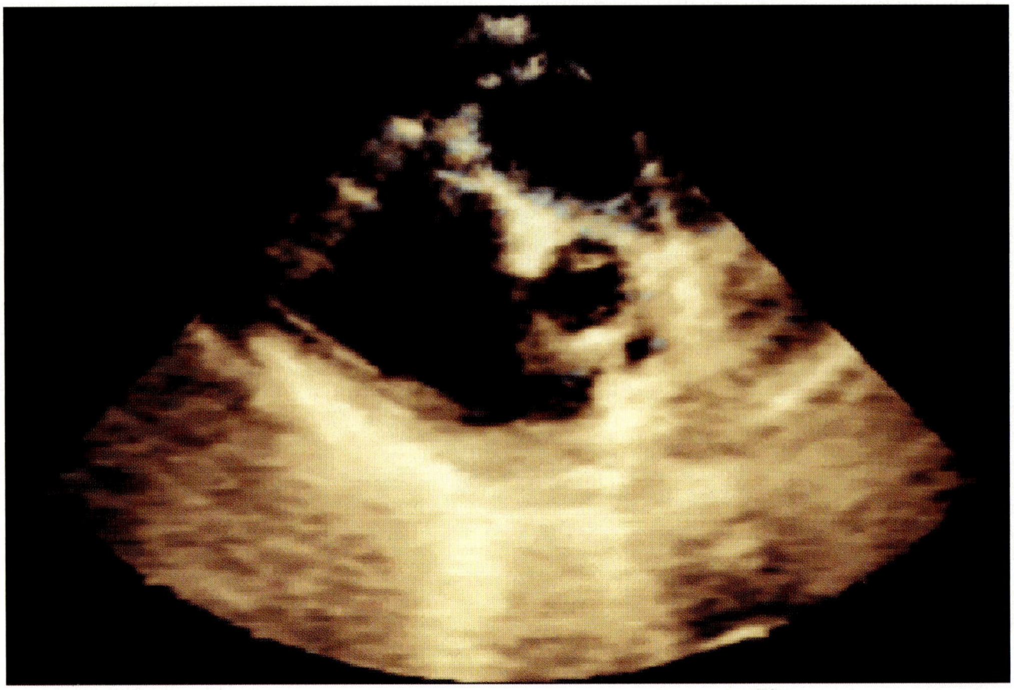

Figure 11: A case of pulmonary atresia

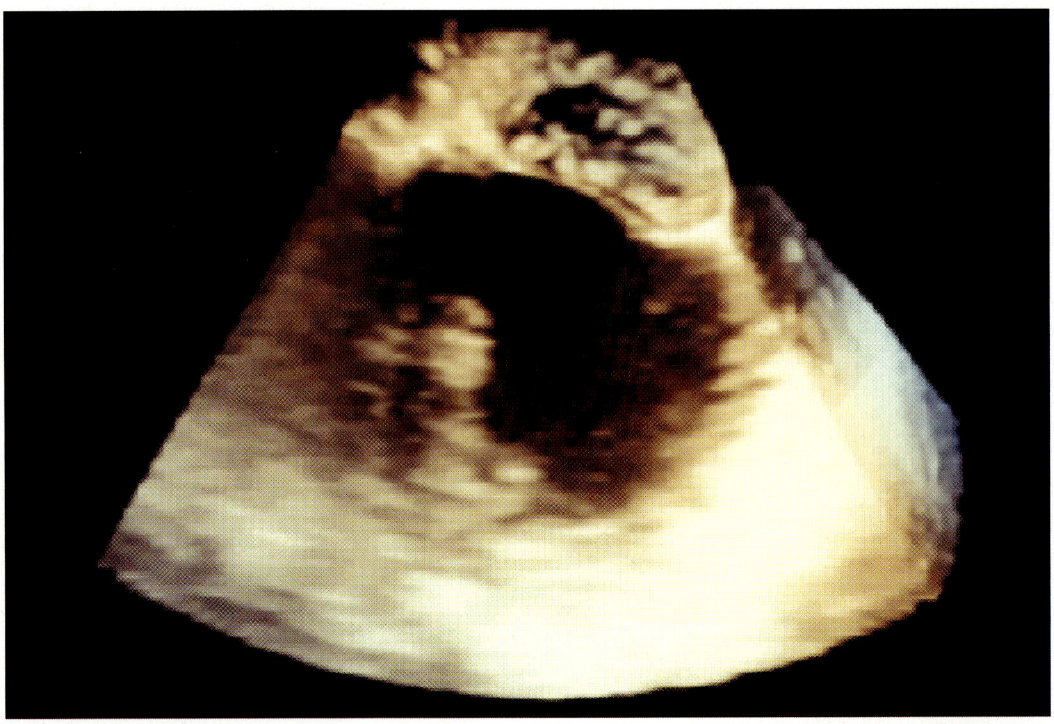

Figure 12: 3D Trans Esophageal Echocardiography: Showing sub mitral aneurysm

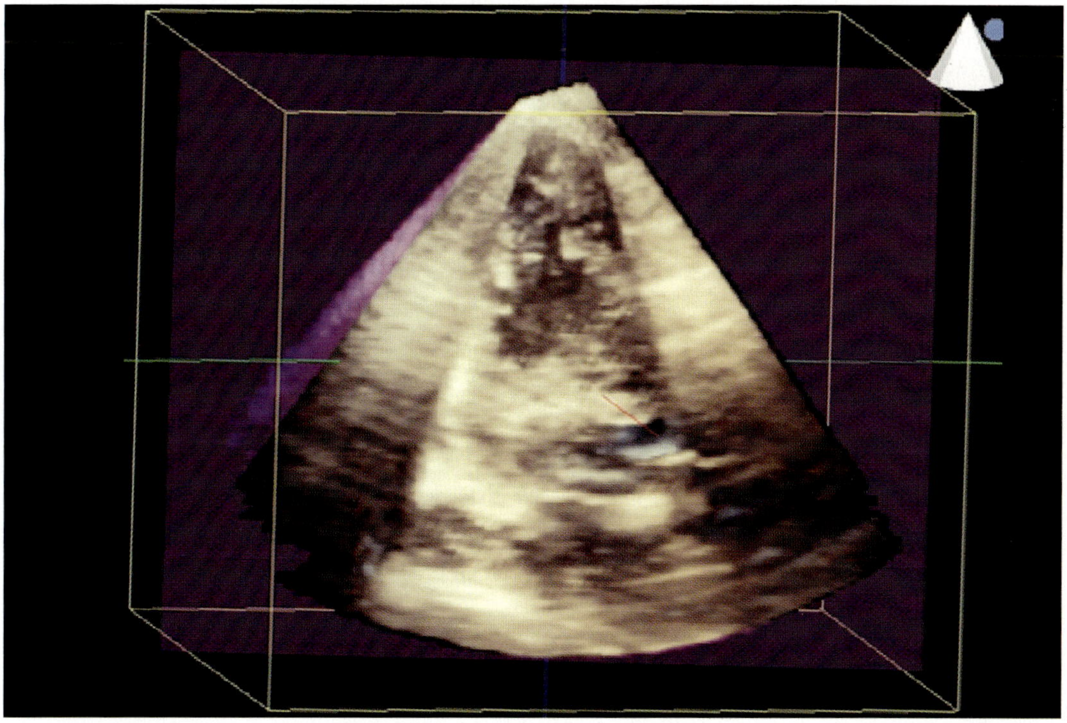

Figure 13: Enface view of VSD

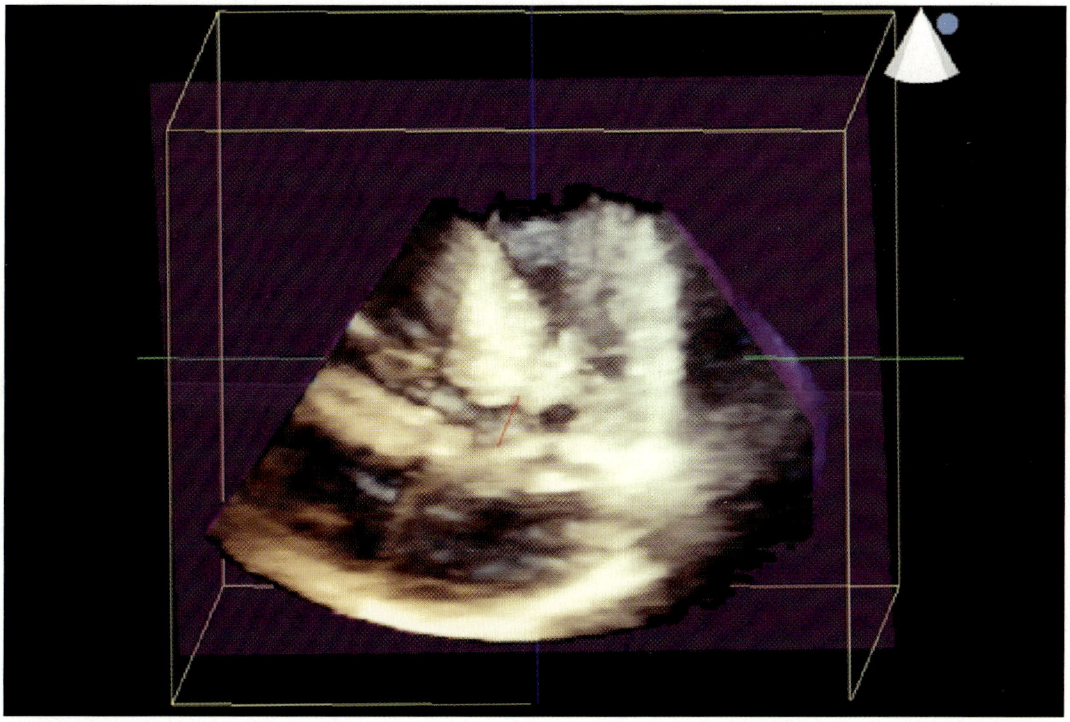

Figure 14: VSD in 3D view

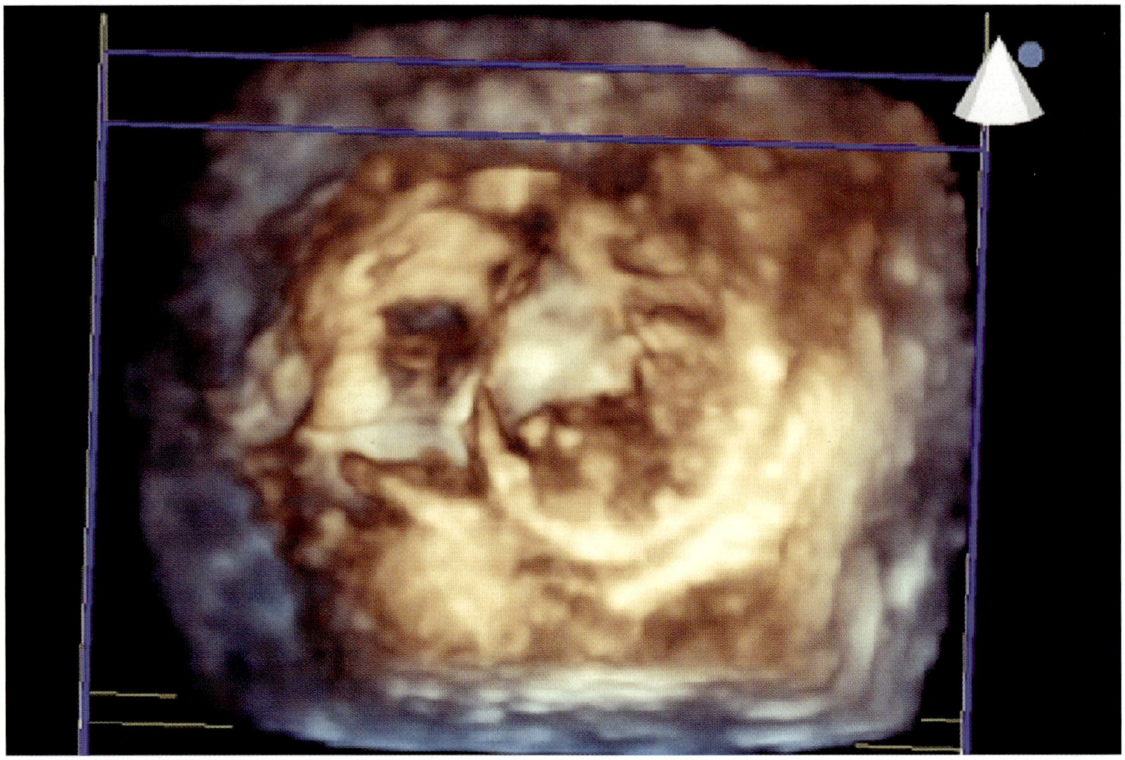

Figure 15: Demonstration of ASD

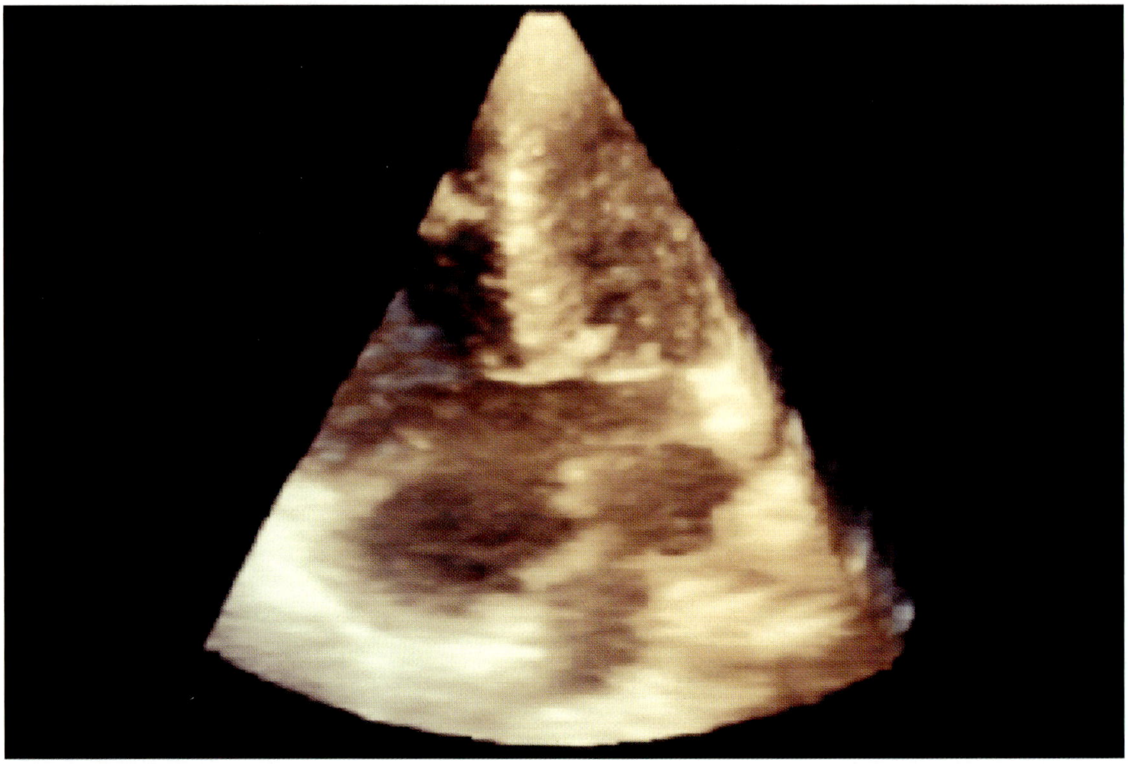

Figure 16: A case of ostium primum ASD

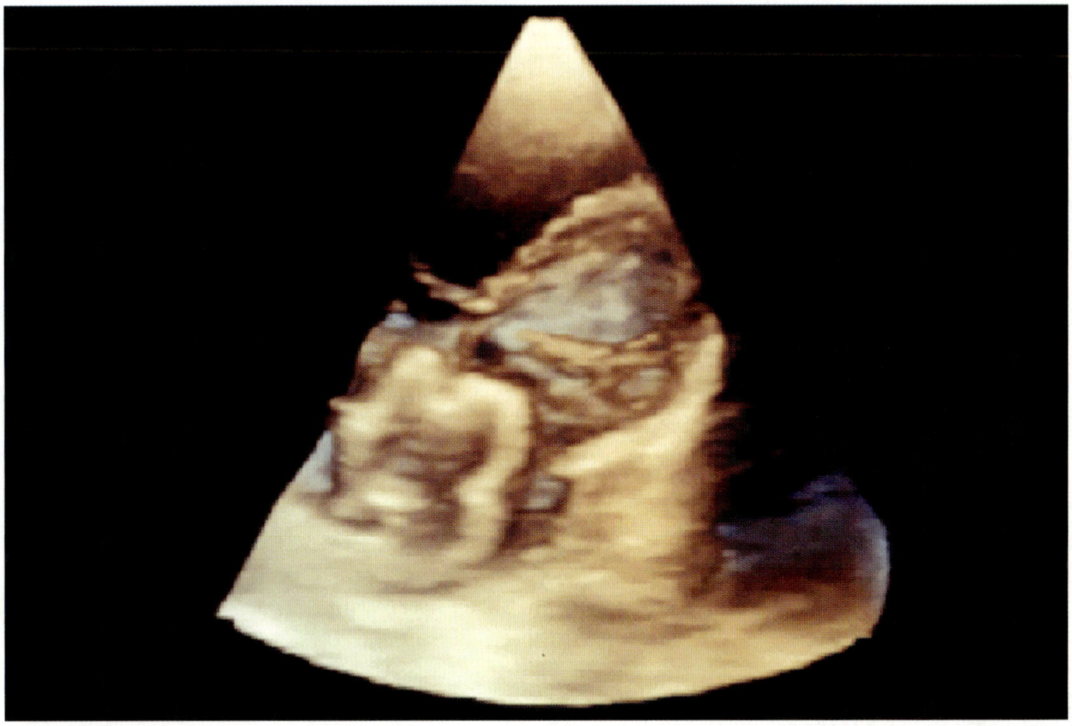

Figure 17: ASD device *in situ*

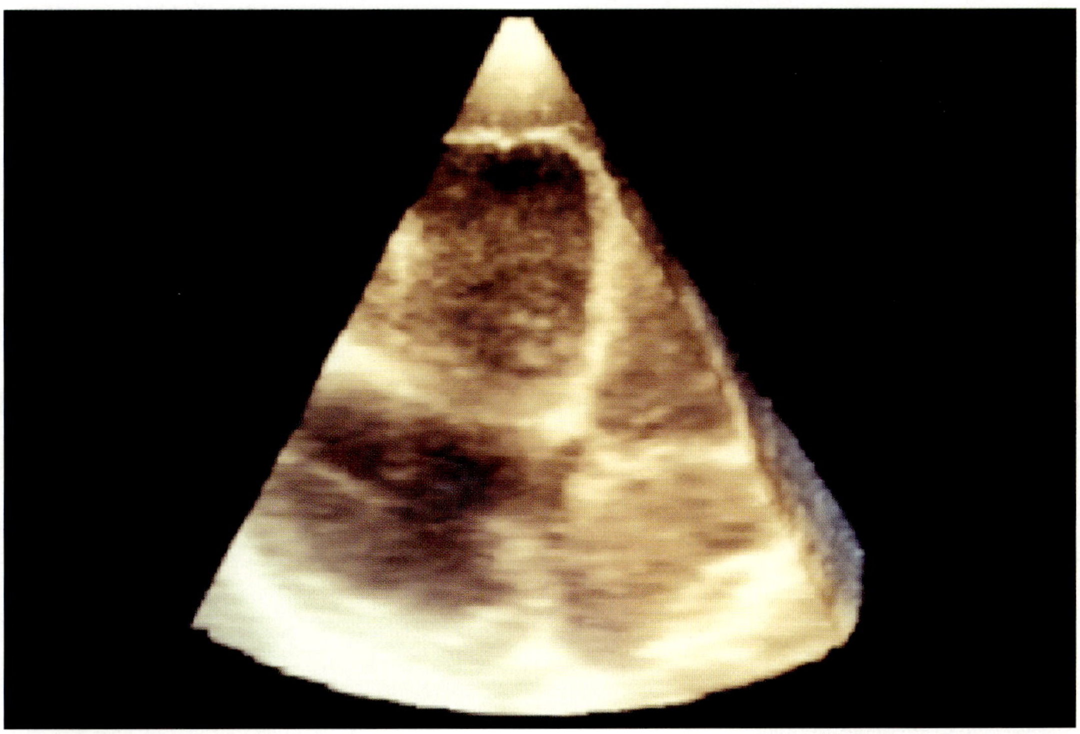

Figure 18: Ebstein's anomaly

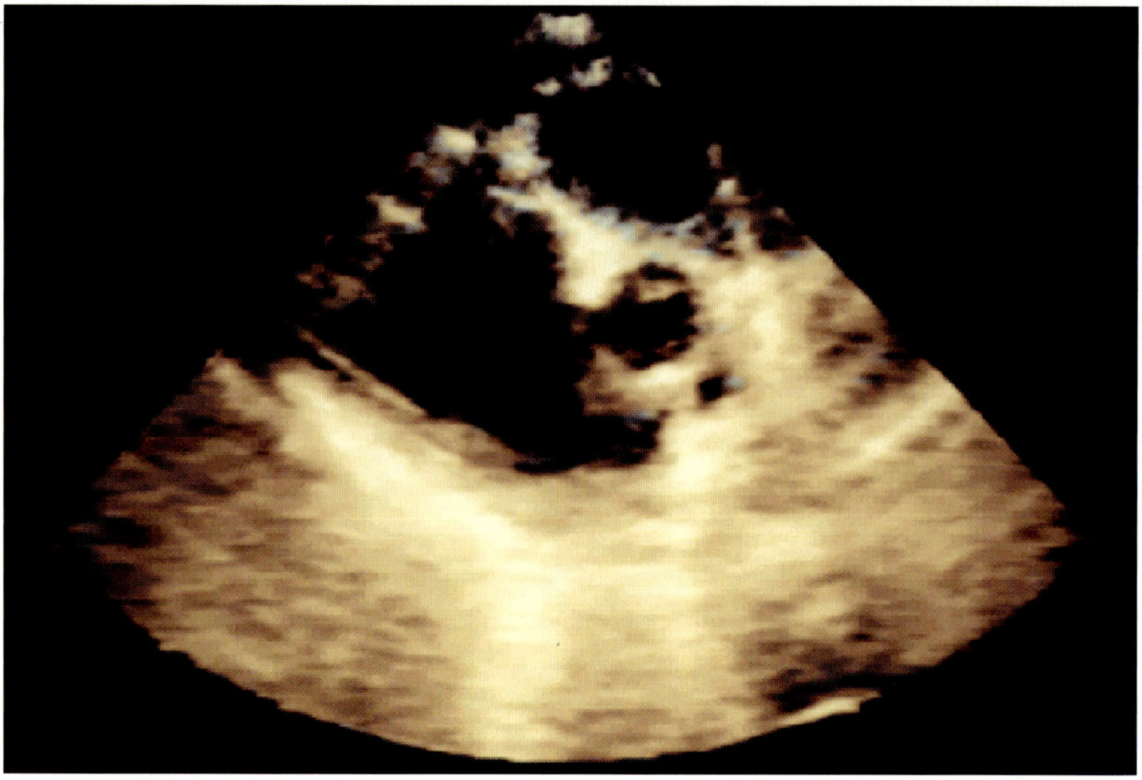

Figure 19: A case of pulmonary atresia

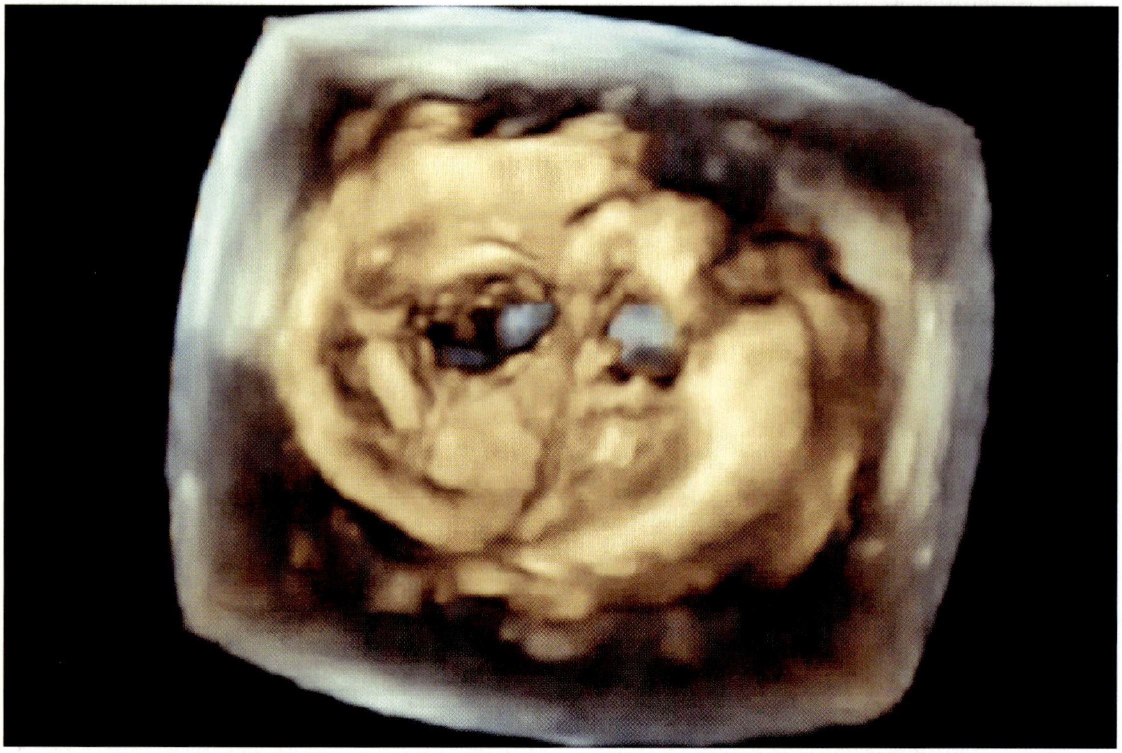

Figure 20: Mitral valve anatomy after PTMC

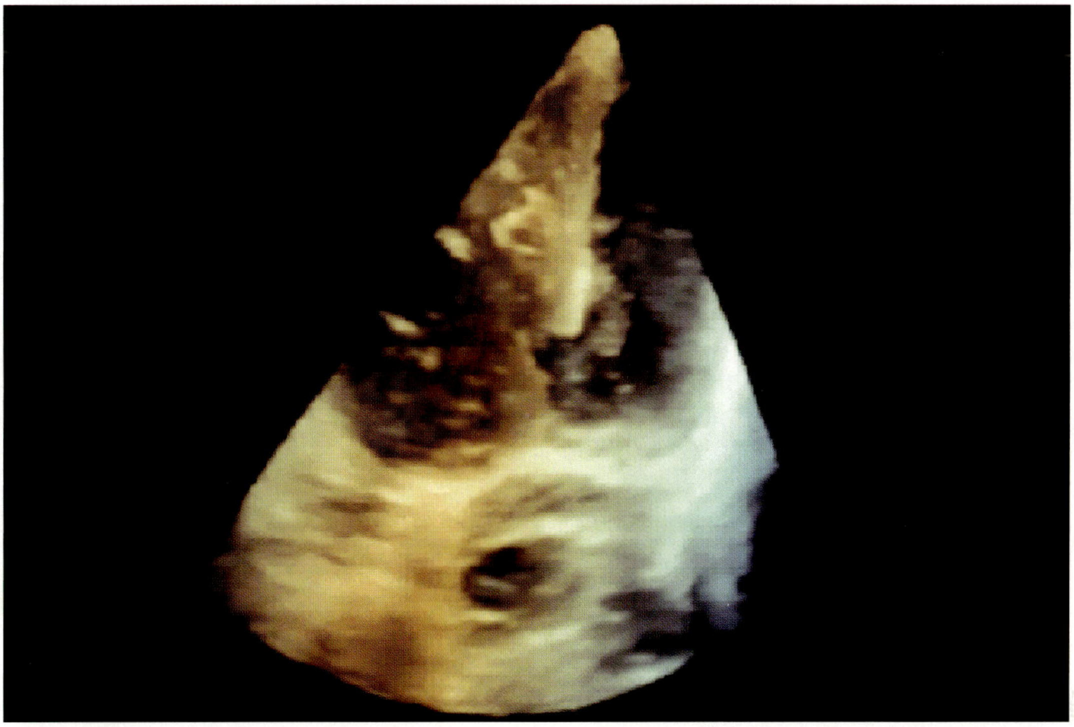

Figure 21: Basal ventricular septal rupture

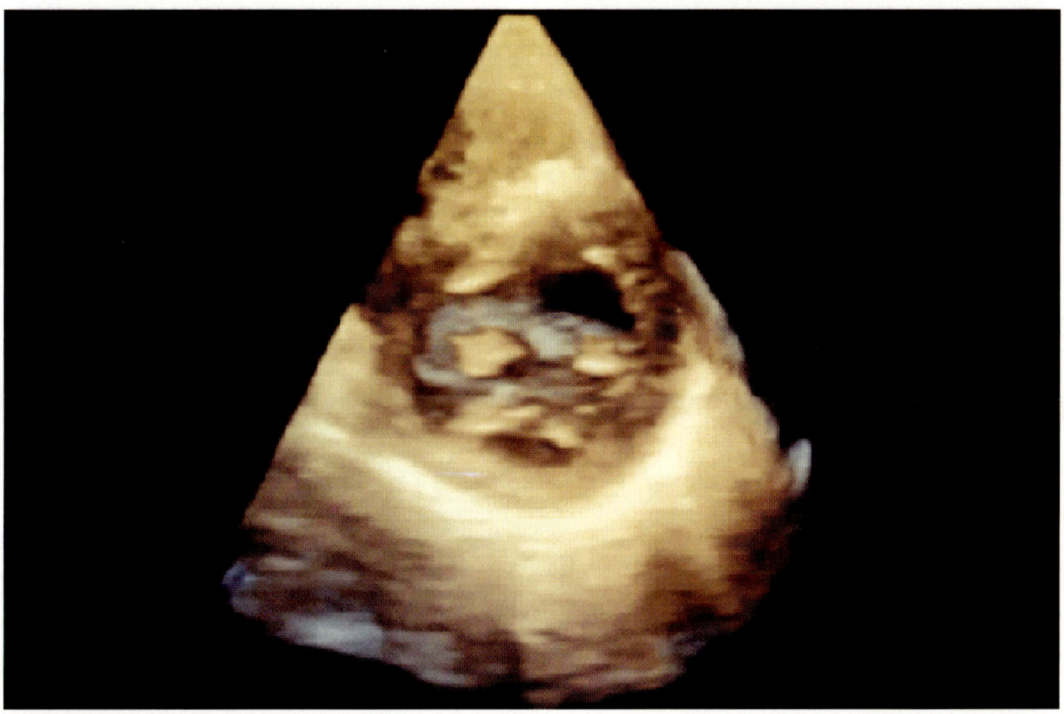

Figure 22: Ventricular septal rupture

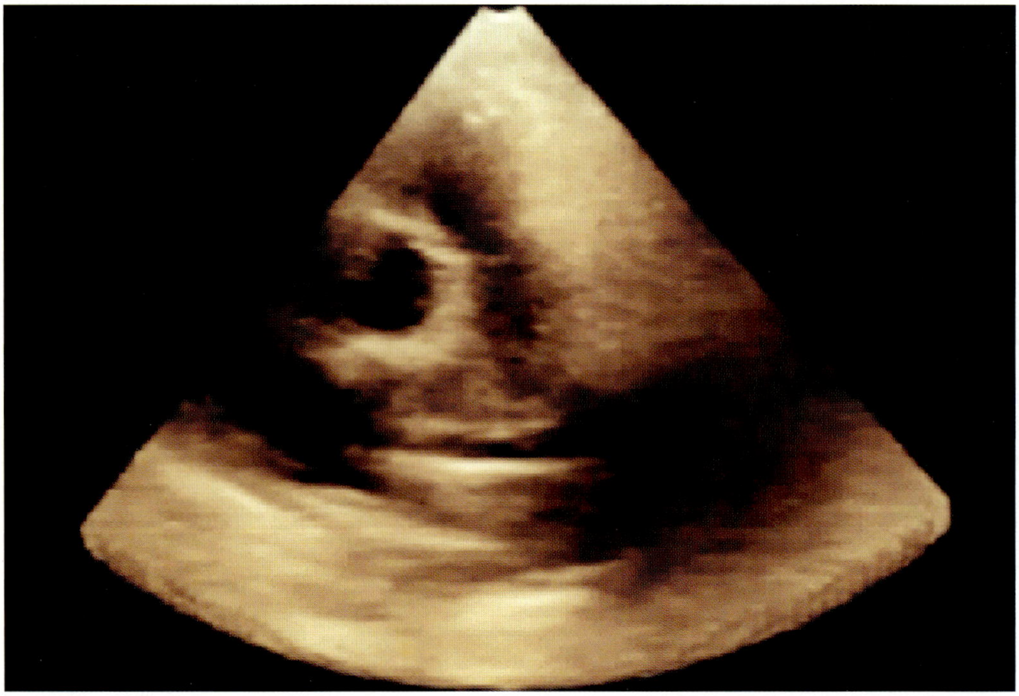

Figure 23: A case of pulmonary thromboembolism with thrombus in MPA

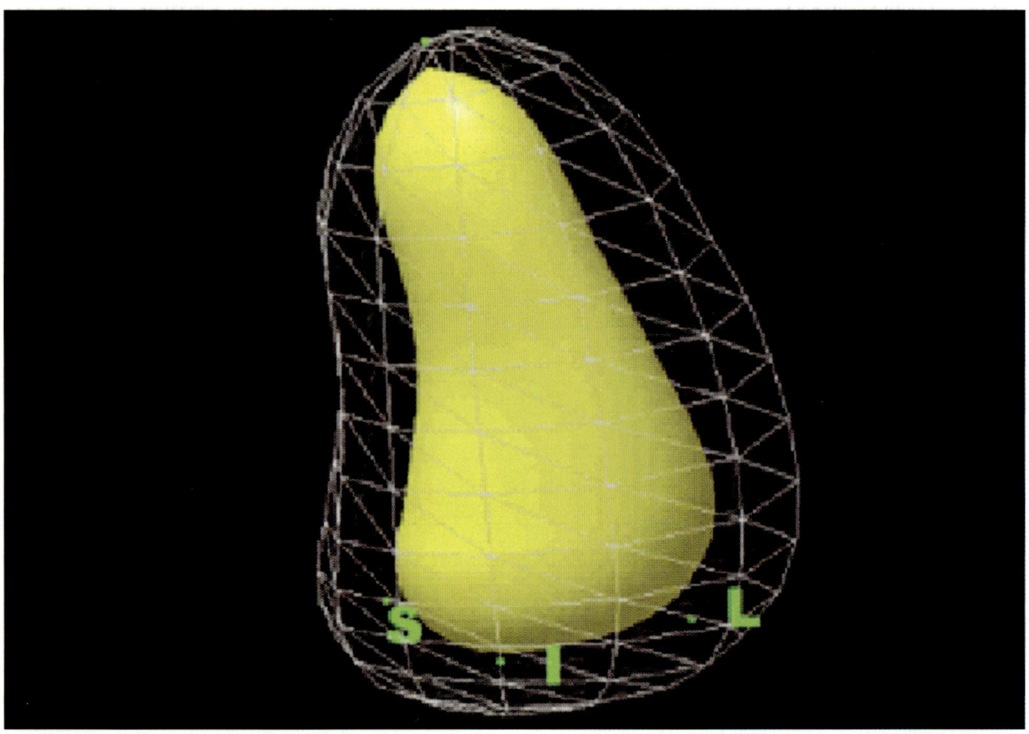

Figure 24: 3D Echo assessment of Left ventricular function : Ejection fraction calculation using Reference Mesh

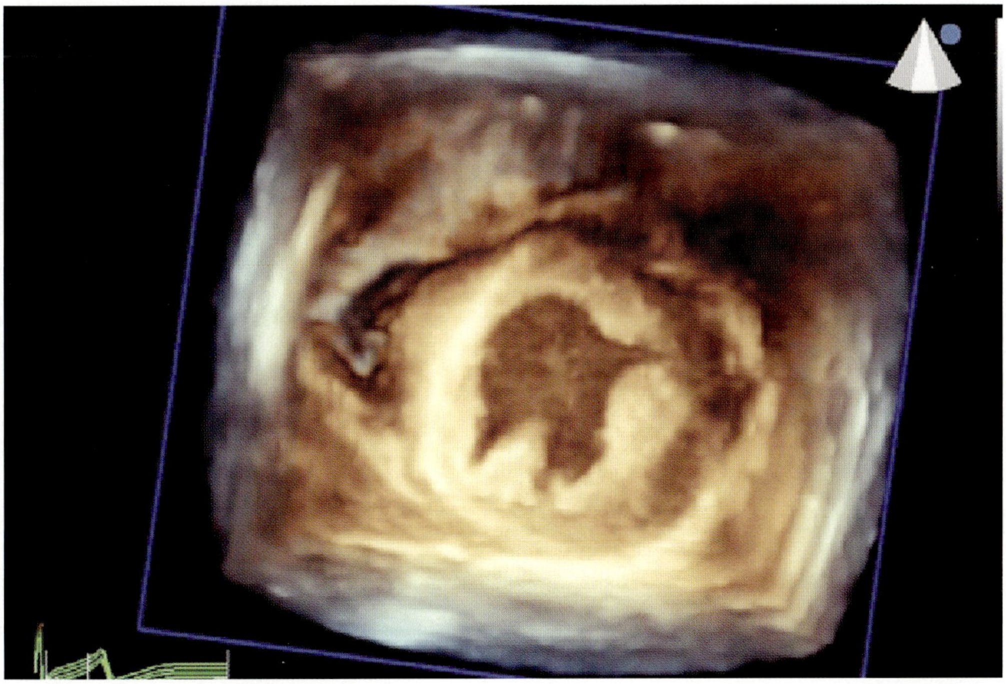

Figure 25: A case of left ventricular hypertrophy

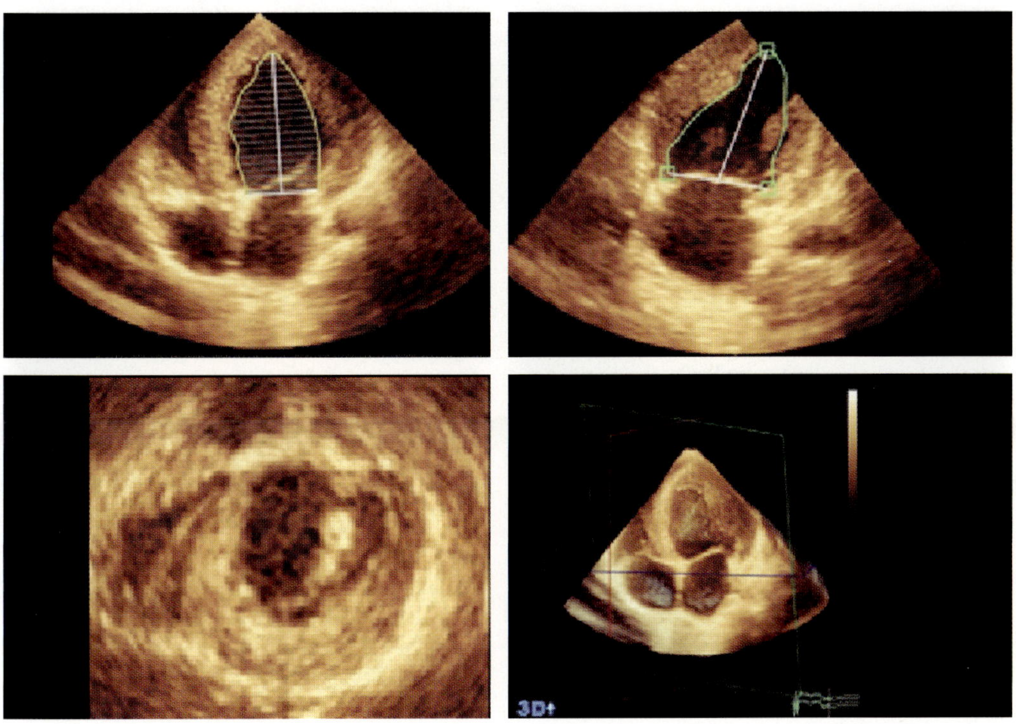

Figure 26: 3D Echo evaluation of a patient with hypertrophic cardiomyopathy

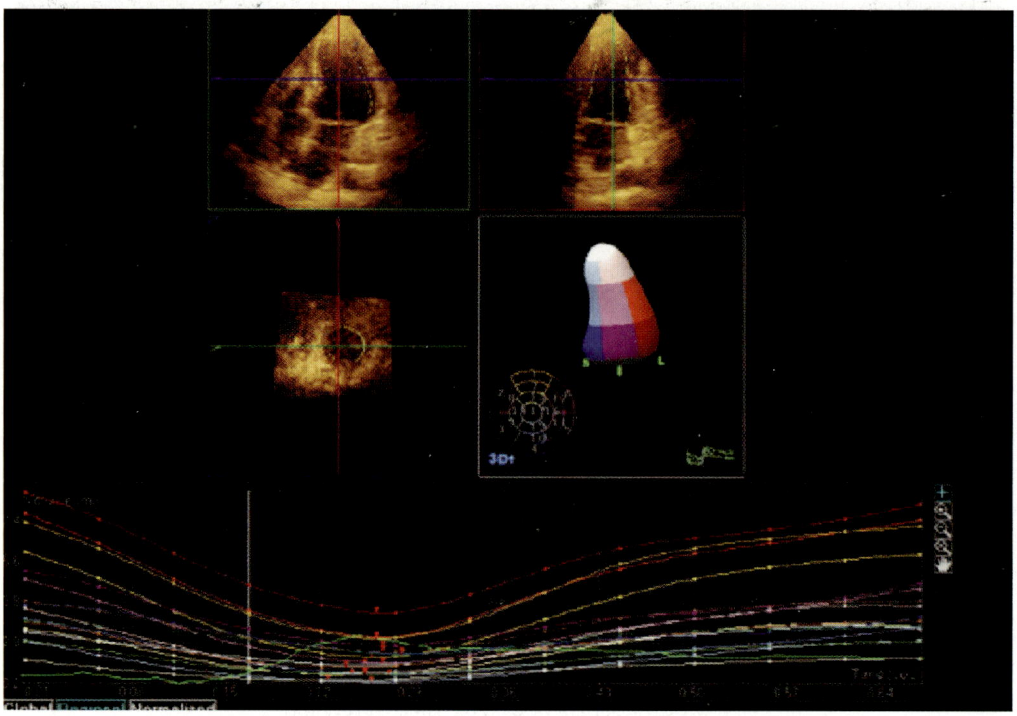

Figure 27: Time volume curves in a patient with acute myocardial infarction

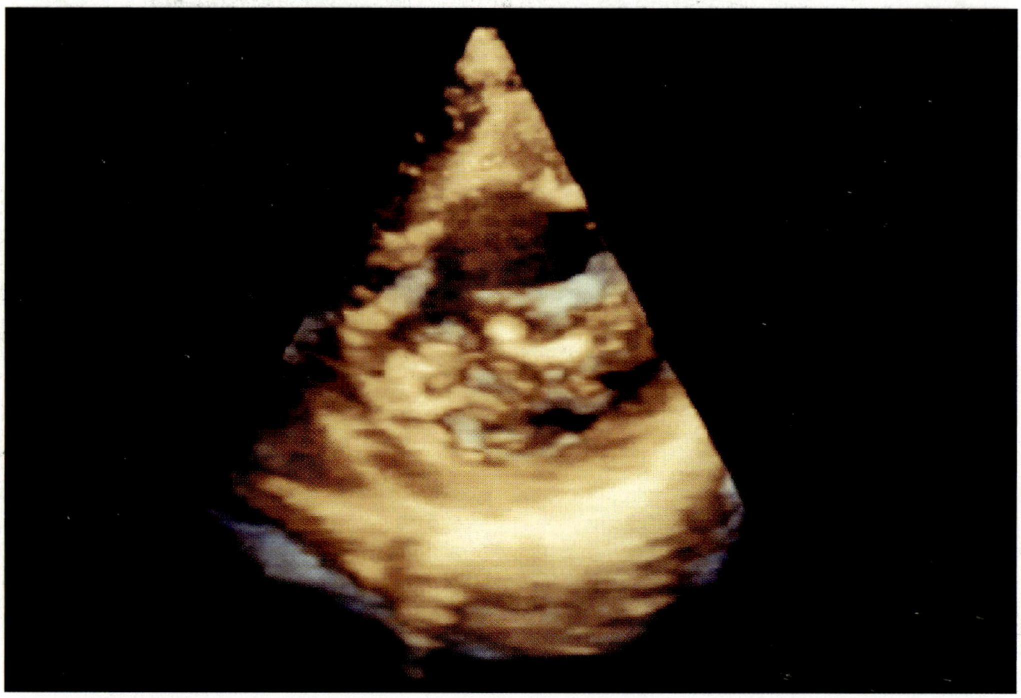

Figure 28: Mitral valve prolapse

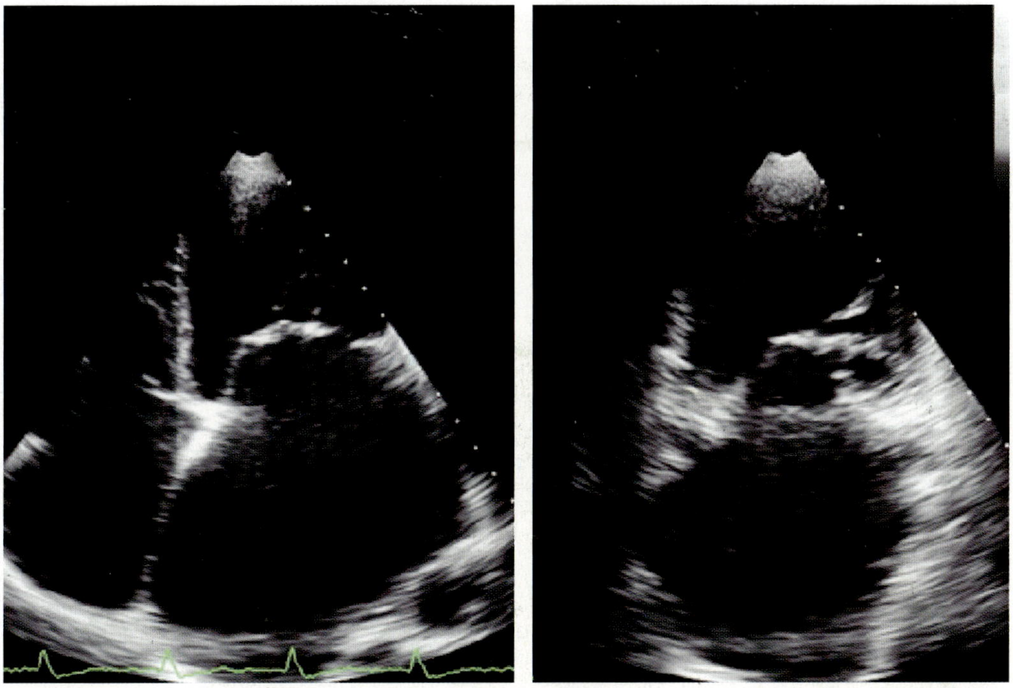

Figure 29: X Plane view : A case of severe MR

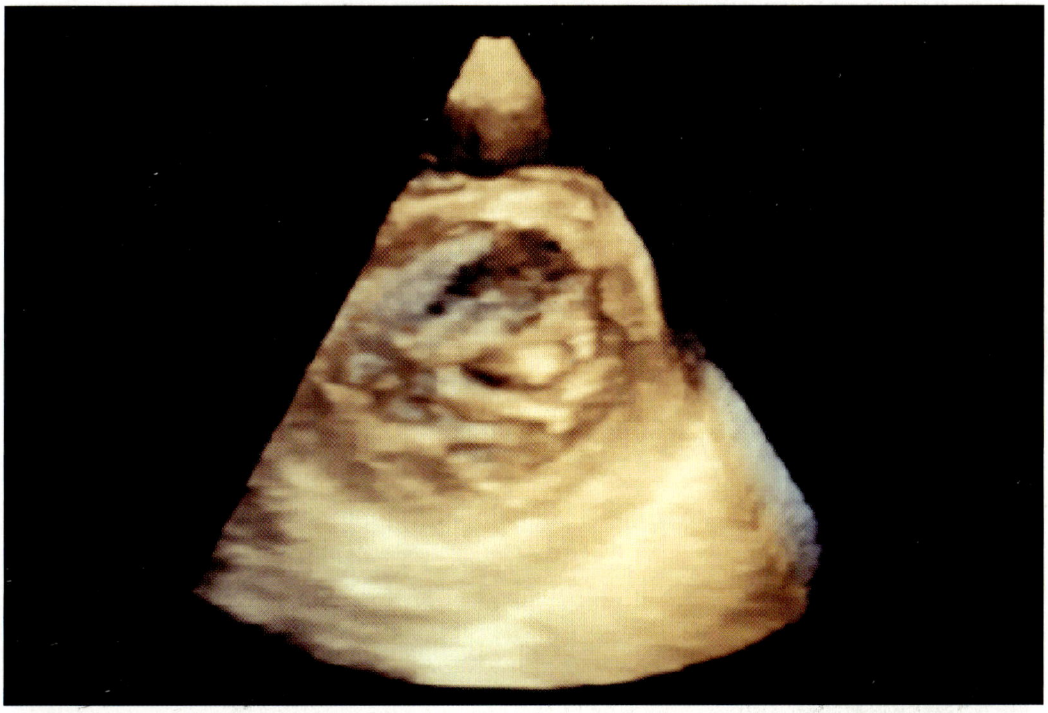

Figure 30: Post mitral valve repair

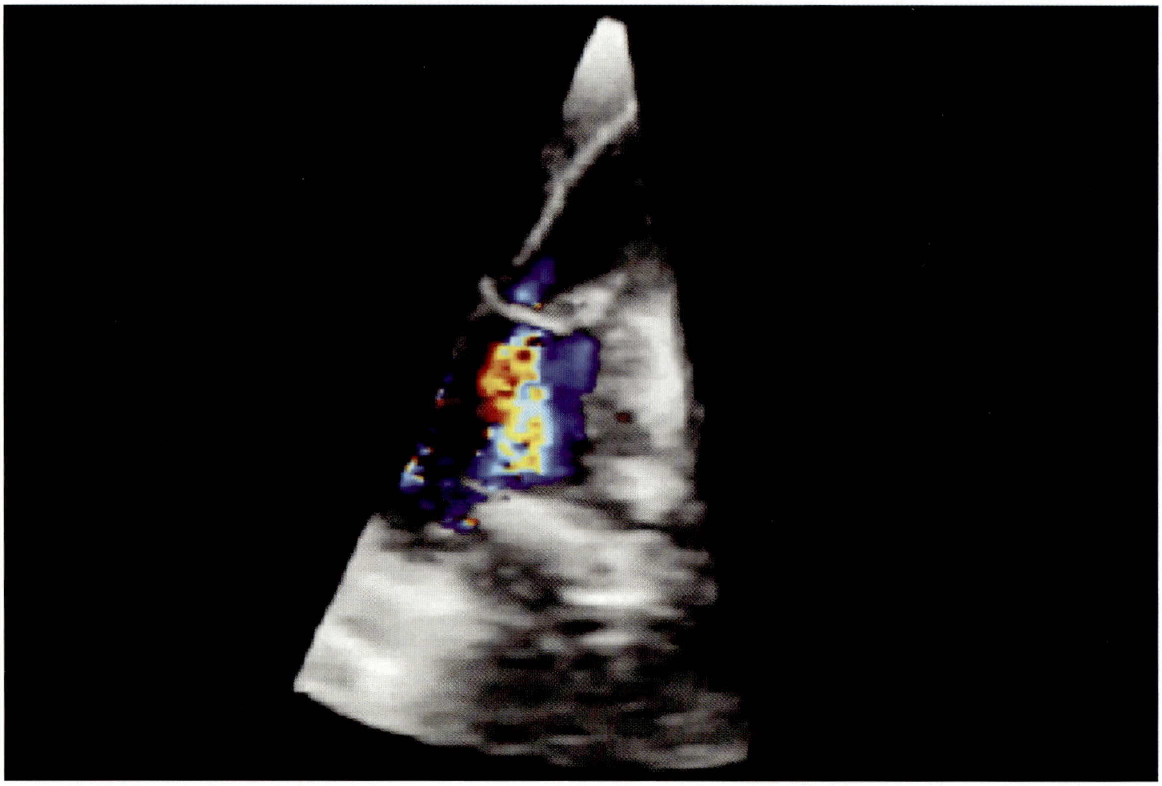

Figure 31: 3D Color Doppler Echocardiography : Mitral regurgitation

Index

Page numbers followed by *f* refer to figure and *t* refer to table

L

M

O

P

Q

R

S

T

U

V